# THE HERBAL HEALING

*Herbalism for Beginners*

## AVA GREEN

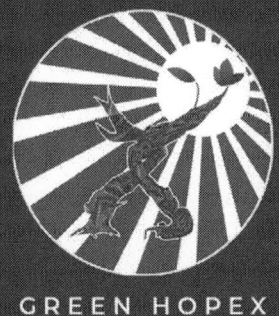

GREEN HOPEX

© **Copyright 2021 Green HopeX – All rights reserved.**

The content contained within this book may not be reproduced, duplicated or transmitted without direct written permission from the author or the publisher.

Under no circumstances will any blame or legal responsibility be held against the publisher, or author, for any damages, reparation, or monetary loss due to the information contained within this book, either directly or indirectly. You are responsible for your own choices, actions, and results.

**Legal Notice:**
This book is copyright protected. This book is only for personal use. You cannot amend, distribute, sell, use, quote or paraphrase any part, or the content within this book, without the consent of the author or publisher.

**Disclaimer Notice:**
Please note the information contained within this document is for educational and entertainment purposes only. All effort has been executed to present accurate, up-to-date, reliable, and complete information. No warranties of any kind are declared or implied. Readers acknowledge that the author is not engaging in the rendering of legal, financial, medical or professional advice. The content within this book has been derived from various sources. Please consult a licensed professional before attempting any techniques outlined in this book.

By reading this document, the reader agrees that under no circumstances is the author responsible for any losses, direct or indirect, which are incurred as a result of the use of the information contained within this document, including, but not limited to, errors, omissions, or inaccuracies.

# Content

Introduction ............................................. 1

The Gifts of Mother Nature ........................ 4

Learning the Ropes .................................. 11
    The Benefits of Herbalism ........................ 11
    The Anatomy of Herbs ............................. 12
    Speaking the Herbal Language .................. 15

The Most Effective Herbs to Know, Grow and Use ... 22
    Your Natural First-Aid Kit ........................ 22
    Other Essential Herbs for the Home Apothecary ... 41

Your Own Medicine Garden and Home Apothecary ... 81
    Harvesting and Processing ....................... 83

Harnessing the Essence of Herbs ................ 89
    Infusions ............................................. 90
    Decoctions .......................................... 93
    Tinctures ............................................ 94
    Syrups ................................................ 97
    Infused Oils ......................................... 99
    Essential Oils ...................................... 103
    Tonic Wines ....................................... 105
    Poultices ........................................... 106
    Ointments ......................................... 108
    Creams ............................................. 109
    Compresses ....................................... 111
    Powders, Capsules, Pills ........................ 112
    Steam Inhalations ............................... 114

Mouth Gargles and Washes . . . . . . . . . . . . . . . . . . . . . 115

# 71 Ailments and Their Herbal Remedies . . . . . . . . . 117

# Handy Herbal Recipes and Mixtures . . . . . . . . . . . 129

# Stay Safe . . . . . . . . . . . . . . . . . . . . . . . . . . . . . . . . . . 134

# Conclusion . . . . . . . . . . . . . . . . . . . . . . . . . . . . . . . . 137

# A Small Favor To Ask . . . . . . . . . . . . . . . . . . . . . . . 138

# References and Further Reading . . . . . . . . . . . . . . . i

## HERB LIST

AGRIMONY ............. 41
ALOE VERA ............ 43
ANGELICA.............. 44
ARNICA ................. 23
BASIL..................... 45
BLACK COHOSH .....47
CALENDULA ...........24
CATNIP...................48
CHAMOMILE ..........50
CHICKWEED ........... 51
COMFREY...............26
DANDELION ...........52
ECHINACEA............27
ELDER ....................54

FENNEL................... 55
FEVERFEW..............29
GARLIC...................30
GINGER ..................56
GINKGO ..................58
GINSENG................59
GOLDENSEAL......... 61
HAWTHORN ...........62
HOPS......................63
LAVENDER.............. 32
LEMON BALM ........65
LICORICE ............... 66
MILK THISTLE .......67
MYRRH................... 33

NETTLE .................. 69
PEPPERMINT .......... 70
ROSEMARY............. 72
SAGE......................73
ST. JOHN'S WORT ....75
TEA TREE................35
THYME ................... 36
TURMERIC.............. 76
VALERIAN............... 38
VERVAIN ................77
WITCH HAZEL ........ 39
YARROW................. 79

## AILMENTS & REMEDIES LIST

#1 Anemia ................................. 117
#2 Anxiety ................................. 117
#3 Acne .................................... 117
#4 Allergies ............................... 118
#5 Asthma ................................ 118
#6 Athlete's Foot........................ 118
#7 Backache ............................. 118
#8 Bee Sting .............................. 118

#9 Bloating ................................. 118
#10 Bronchitis............................. 119
#11 Bruises................................. 119
#12 Burns.................................. 119
#13 Chapped Lips ...................... 119
#14 Canker Sore......................... 119
#15 Chickenpox.......................... 119
#16 Cold...................................120

#17 Cold Sore............................. 120
#18 Colic ................................... 120
#19 Conjunctivitis ..................... 120
#20 Constipation....................... 120
#21 Cough................................. 120
#22 Dandruff ............................ 120
#23 Diaper Rash ....................... 121
#24 Diarrhea ............................. 121
#25 Digestive Inflammation Including GERD (Gastroesophageal Reflux Disease) ........................... 121
#26 Earache............................... 121
#27 Eczema............................... 121
#28 Fatigue ............................... 121
#29 Fever.................................. 122
#31 Fractures............................ 122
#32 Gastritis.............................. 122
#33 Gingivitis (Gum Inflammation)........................................... 122
#34 Hair Loss ............................ 122
#35 Halitosis (Bad Breath) ..... 122
#36 Hangover ...........................123
#37 Headache ..........................123
#38 Hemorrhoids .....................123
#39 High Blood Pressure..........123
#40 Hives .................................123
#41 Indigestion........................123
#42 Insect Bites .......................123
#43 Insomnia............................ 124
#44 Liver Infections.................. 124
#45 Menopause ....................... 124
#46 Mental Focus..................... 124
#47 Muscle Cramps.................. 124
#48 Nausea .............................. 124
#49 Period Pain........................ 124
#50 Premenstrual Syndrome (PMS) ......................................... 124
#51 Psoriasis .............................125

#52 Rheumatoid Arthritis........... 125
#53 Shingles................................ 125
#54 Sinus Infection ..................... 125
#55 Skin Tags.............................. 125
#56 Sore Muscles........................126
#57 Sore Throat..........................126
#58 Sprains .................................126
#59 Stiff Joints............................126
#60 Stomach Spasms .................126
#61 Stress....................................126
#62 Sunburn................................126
#63 Swelling and Fluid Retention ..................................................126
#64 Tongue Ulcers ...................... 127
#65 Tonsillitis.............................. 127
#66 Travel Sickness .................... 127
#67 Urinary Tract Infection (UTI) .................................................. 127
#68 Varicose Veins ..................... 127
#69 Warts................................... 127
#70 Wounds ............................... 127
#71 Yeast Infection.....................128

# SPECIAL BONUS!

## Want this book for free?

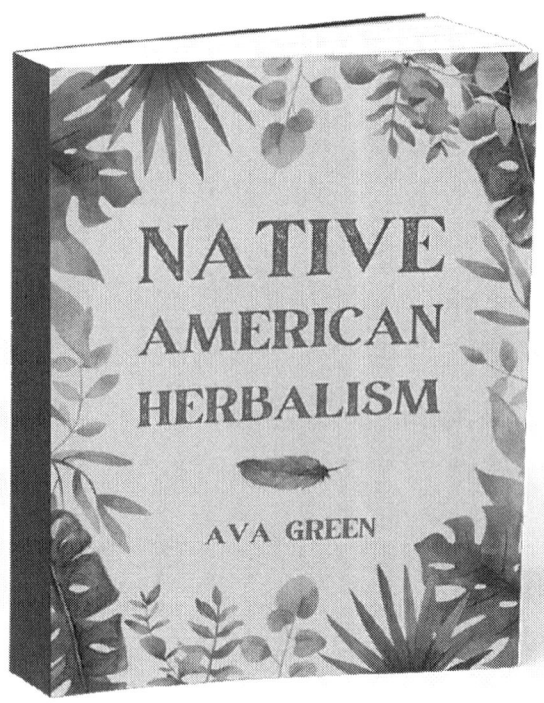

Get FREE unlimited access to it and all my new books by joining our Fan Jam!

Scan with your camera to join!

# Introduction

How much money does the average developed country spend on healthcare each year? Hundreds of billions; trillions even. The sum for most first-world countries is nearly out of the realm of our understanding and yet, most of the population struggles to stay healthy. We live on a constant adrenaline rush, heading to work, or to school. We are on the go and, while we live our busy lives, we allow toxins in. We don't have time to be selective about what goes into our bodies, and we tend to pop a pill whenever we need to forget about our discomfort. The result of this is a high level of ambivalence towards taking pills and an increased dependence on such drugs.

Undoubtedly, we need conventional Western medicine. Many serious illnesses require a drug-based approach to keep us enlivened and energized. But that doesn't mean that we should rely on it blindly. Before modern medicine, people were living their lives in a wholesome and healthy way. There were lethal diseases that medicinal plants couldn't battle, of course, but we can embrace conventional medicine in those situations. For everything else, let's find the cure in the natural world!

Over the last couple of decades, public awareness of herbal medicine has skyrocketed. People are slowly regaining trust in nature and realizing that our role intertwines with the planet's existence. We are creatures of the Earth. Handle her carefully and she will care for you in return.

Herbs are packed with active constituents that can

stimulate, support, restrain, and retrain different parts of our bodies, restoring their normal function. When used wisely, plants with therapeutic properties can work in harmony with our bodies to produce balanced health.

There are thousands of therapeutic plants, each with the ability to address and heal certain health issues. This book covers 40 of the most effective and commonly used ones, to give you a decent nudge in the right direction. Start with these herbs, and you boast hundreds of options for natural treatments in the case of most health troubles. In this book, you will also find 71 aliments and their corresponding remedies. These are merely shadows on the wall of all the wonderful uses for medicinal plants.

With 15 different extraction methods explained in detail, and bonus recipes that will help you start your healing journey right away, this will be your go-to herbal source whenever you feel like whipping up a natural cure. From how to harvest, extract, preserve, and store the herbs and their remedies, to when, and how to use them, I am sharing my ultimate secrets about the ancient art of herbal healing with every aspiring herbalist.

No fancy tools are needed, no extensive knowledge of biology required; all you need for this healing journey is the willingness to take it! Follow the advice wisely and safely, and a hale and hearty living is guaranteed

## Note before reading

This book offers knowledge on how to extract medicinal herbs and make herbal remedies to address many health issues. It is a beginner-friendly guide, free of heavy and complex terminology, offering a simple and step-by-step approach to herbalism.

It is not, by any means, an herbal encyclopedia or an advanced book for well-seasoned herbalists.

The book is written by an experienced and knowledgeable herbalism enthusiast, not a physician. No parts of this book are meant to replace the advice of a medical professional. Use the herbs with caution and refer to the safety sections first. Always research the herbs well before using them, and consult with your physician for any uncertainties.

The author of this book cannot guarantee the effect of the remedies, as we all have unique conditions and requirements. The author cannot be held accountable for any injuries, misinterpretations, improper use, possible side effects or any adverse consequences.

# The Gifts of Mother Nature

**W**hen I first began to explore the benefits of herbal medicine, I started with the basics – lavender, chamomile, calendula, garlic. I had grown up watching my nana and mother do wonders with the herbs from our backyard. To me, they had seemed like magicians mixing up potions. The magic of these plants was instilled in me young. As I grew, my curiosity about the world of natural remedies expanded and I actually gave this medicine a shot when I got married. I planted my own garden. Now I have more than 30 different medicinal plants always at my fingertips, and a whole pantry stocked with remedies that help me fight diseases and keep illnesses at bay.

I was lucky enough to become familiarized with herbal healing from a very young age, so I didn't approach it with skepticism. But for those who think that the herbalism boom is nothing more than taking Instagram-worthy shots of colorful dried plants, or that herbal potions are only for big-nosed witches, allow me to show you a more accurate picture of the path to herbal healing.

Herbal healing may have been born out of necessity but even in this modern era we still walk the path paved by our ancestors. Conventional medicine may be needed in some cases, but we often forget that people in the past relied solely on what Mother Nature had to offer. And with antibiotics and other medical treatments sometimes having negative effects, therapeutic herbs are regaining the trust they lost. So many pathogens are becoming resistant to chemically loaded drugs.

As far as we know, Mother Nature has given us 50,000 to 70,000 plants with therapeutic properties; small shrubs, lichens, tiny fungi, green mosses, tall trees. It is up to us, the modern practitioners, to discover these medicinal herbs and learn how to extract their healing properties in safe and effective ways. And people have been doing that since the dawn of humanity. Every culture in the world has its own herbal traditions, whether sensible or magical, and a unique connection to nature: the oldest medicine.

## Europe

Europe's herbalism history was mainly influenced by Asian practices but can be traced back to Hippocrates, an Ancient Greek philosopher, who lived from 460 –377 BC. By classifying the herbs as hot, dry, cold, or moist, Hippocrates set the foundation of traditional herbal healing. His "four humors" represented the four bodily fluids (phlegm, blood, yellow bile, and black bile) and how they corresponded with the four elements of nature (water, fire, air, and earth).

Hippocrates developed a base of healing in Greece, and herbalism quickly took over the Earth's cradle. Greece's major urban centers soon came along for the ride. Rome happily started to learn about the properties of herbal medicine. The majority of traditional knowledge of herbalism in Rome actually came from Dioscorides, who was a Roman army surgeon from AD 40–90. After observing 600 plants, he wrote his *De Materia Medica*, which further shed light on the use of plants for therapeutic purposes.

Although folk medicine was handed down from one generation to the next, European herbalism reached its apex in the 15th century, thanks to the invention of printing. In the following centuries, many herbalists managed to print herbal catalogs, in various languages, and to share their application secrets with the public. The most notable herbal reference books come from two English herbalists. John Gerard's novel *The Herbail* (1597), and Nicholas Culpeper's *The English Physitian* (1652) are the gems of herbalism in Europe. Ever since their publication, they have been providing valuable knowledge and herbal information for anyone looking to explore (or exploit) the gifts of Mother Nature.

With the rise of importation in the 17th and 18th centuries, foreign herbs were introduced into Europe. European herbalists now had the chance to expand their knowledge and improve practices. And they did so with vigor! In the 18th century, almost 70% of all medicinal plants used in Europe were imported.

When conventional medicine saw a rise in popularity, herbalism was slowly but surely cast aside. Once the pharmaceutical monopoly spread across Europe, it became illegal to practice herbalism without a special medical certificate. It was only four decades ago that herbalism started to regain its glory. Now there are many modern practitioners of herbal medicine and, in some European countries, natural remedies are routinely prescribed.

### The Middle East and India

If you're into herbalism, then you've probably heard of *Ayurveda medicine.* Ayurveda is the oldest Middle Eastern and Indian healing system. It stretches way beyond simple treatment, into the realms of religion, philosophy, and science. These are considered the main components of one's being. At its core, the use of therapeutic herbs, yoga, meditation, and other practices help one reach total harmony.

This ancient practice has used medicinal plants, such as turmeric, since 4,000 BC. Early common people worked with herbal medicine for many generations, but the first official Ayurvedic school was founded in 400 BC by Punarvasu Atreya. This opened up a whole world of herbal healing for the doctors of old. Most herbs and healing minerals were discovered by the popular ancient Indian herbalists Charaka and Sushurta, in the first millennium BC.

This unique holistic approach is known to be one of the oldest medicinal practices. With Buddhism's rise, from 563–483 BC, and onward, Ayurveda became known throughout Asia, and would eventually spread to most of the developed world.

Although the British banned Ayurveda completely in the 19th century, by the time India became independent there were many herbalists ready to resurrect this healing approach. Since 1947, Ayurveda has been known as a valid and effective natural treatment system throughout the world.

## China and Southeast Asia

China is the only country in the world that can brag about having an ancient herbal healing tradition that is as appreciated by people as is conventional Western medicine. Although Chinese folk medicine has been around since humans first began wandering through Asia, their traditional herbalism dates from sometime around 200 BC. The first ideas are recorded in the Chinese manuscript, *Yellow Emperor's Classic of Internal Medicine*. The main concepts throughout the book teach that life is at the mercy of the natural laws.

Traditional Chinese Medicine (TCM) has two systems: one is based on the principles of *yin* and *yang*, and the other on the five elements (wood, fire, water, earth, and metal). The principles of *yin* and *yang* state that everything has a complementary opposite; light and dark, and good and evil. The five-element system describes how our internal organs are classified and connected. The two TCM branches developed separately, and five-element healing wasn't born until sometime between the years 960–1279, during the Song dynasty.

Chinese herbalism is quite unique. Instead of just trying to cure the symptoms, a TCM practitioner seeks to find what causes the disharmony in the body. It is a much more effective approach to healing because it goes beyond symptom relief. For instance, if you catch a cold, a Chinese herbal practitioner will not just prescribe you a tincture or infusion to help you get better. He or she will observe your whole being to find out why your body hasn't adjusted well to the external factors such as wind and temperature.

Ancient Chinese medicine has greatly influenced the rest of southeast Asia, mostly Japan and Korea. The traditional Japanese medicine called *Kampoh* dates from the 5th century. This form of medicine was inspired by TCM. In Korea, herbal remedies are very similar to those used in traditional Chinese medicine.

Although TCM is now widely recognized and used for healing, it mostly addresses chronic conditions. For more serious and acute illnesses, it is replaced with conventional Western medicine, even in China.

## Africa

The oldest preserved medical record in Africa is the Ebers Papyrus, which dates back to around 1550 BC. Although it is now believed to have been nothing more than a copy of previous medical collections, it clearly shows us that herbs have been used for their therapeutic properties since ancient times in Africa. This text refers to over 700 medicinal herbs and includes more than 870 different prescriptions for unique conditions.

Although most of the herbal practices were suppressed during colonial times, many traditional African healers are well-respected throughout the world today. Colonizers attempted many times to wipe out the culture of herbal practice in Africa, but today herbal remedies are widely available both in urban and rural settings. There are many remote places on the continent that have never changed their practices. Even today, African people living in far-flung rural areas, away from hospitals and conventional medical care, depend solely on their herbal remedies. They are used for chronic, simple, and serious or life-threatening conditions.

## Australia and New Zealand

Aboriginal Australians settled the island continent over 60,000 years ago and possibly have the oldest and richest herbal tradition of any culture in the world. Disastrously, with the arrival of European settlers and the disruption of Aboriginal life, much of the knowledge of their healing practices vanished into a deep, forgotten well. However, bush medicine is still used in parts of Australia, and there are current efforts to record these traditions in written form. There are still many indigenous plants, like Eucalyptus, that we use and understand, thanks to Aboriginal knowledge and practices.

Similarly, after the Maori arrived in New Zealand, some 1000 years ago, they developed their own medicinal uses for some of the indigenous plants. For example, they used *Manuka* to treat skin diseases, colds, and as a sedative. Today we also know *Manuka* as a type of tea tree (*Leptospermum scoparium*), and its oil is prized as an herbal remedy. Some of our knowledge of the ways in which Maori used medicinal plants comes from the records written by the early European settlers and missionaries.

In the last 200 years, plants from Australia and New Zealand have become part of herbal medicine throughout the world. After 1989, when the Therapeutic Goods Act (an act of Australian legislation) was passed, Australia and New Zealand started developing their herbal medicine industry, offering many natural, over-the-counter alternatives. They also commenced with commercial cultivation of therapeutic herbs, and even offer university training for aspiring practitioners.

**North and Central America**

The history of herbalism in North America stems from rural practices in Central America. The first American evidence of these medical cures is *The Badianus Manuscript* from 1552. It is an Aztec list of Mexican herbs used for healing purposes.

Shamanism, a religious practice that involves interacting with spirits, is closely tied to herbal healing in Central America. What is so intriguing about American herbalism is that throughout the northern and southern continents, from Canada to Chile, native people believed herbs to be bursting with spiritual energy, and packed with healing powers.

When European settlers arrived in North America, in the 17th century, they slowly realized the nature of these practices. The native people were thought to be primitive but, in fact, their herbal medicine was effective. Settlers discovered they could learn from these people and thus a knot was tied between Native American and Western herbalism. This knot inspired Dr. Wooster Beech to found Eclecticism in the 1830s, and combine herbal tradition with new scientific knowledge. By 1909, there were over 8,000 followers and practitioners of the new movement.

The practice of herbal medicine in the United States started declining in the early 20th century due to the fact that plants couldn't be patented. This meant that all pharmaceutical companies could develop herbal medicines, so competition was stiff and profits decreased. The rich and powerful threw their money behind allopathic (conventional) medical schools and the others slowly died. Practicing doctors practiced what they were taught so, once there were only allopathic schools, herbal knowledge lost favor. When supportive legislation was passed in 1994, herbalism in America let out a whoop of delight and began its journey back to popularity. In the past couple of decades, North American people have started using herbs extensively for healing purposes, and the number of herbal practitioners throughout the continent is growing by the day.

**South America**

When thinking of South American herbalism, the first things that come to mind are rituals, sacrifices, and magic. South America is known to have many hallucinogenic plants that allowed its native people to "communicate" with spirits. But beyond shamanism, there is a wide variety of different herbal practices and traditions throughout the continent. From the Amazon region to the city of Rio de Janeiro, each South American culture is dominated by specific plants and their usages. Thanks to the abundance of thick rainforests, South America holds the title of the continent with the most mysterious, unexplained, and unexplored medicinal potential.

With the Spanish conquests in the 16th century, Europeans started exporting plants to Europe. Soon after this, native South American herbal traditions and secret remedies spread throughout the world. Today, in South America, herbal practitioners combine native and Western methods of healing.

Tragically, South American herbalism, and many of the native medicinal plants, are under threat of becoming extinct as, every year, more of the rainforests are cut down or further exploited by money-hungry corporations.

Irrespective of herbalism's history, today there is a growing interest in medicinal plants throughout the world. As the non-selective use of conventional drugs is on the rise, the effects that these drugs have on diseases has started to decrease. This forces us to look for alternative treatments to complement the conventional drugs, so that we can have these drugs as a reserve to use only when necessary. And herbalism offers just that. Read on to see exactly how you can benefit from this natural approach to healing.

# Learning the Ropes

You may be tempted to skip this chapter and get straight to the nitty-gritty of using herbs for medicinal purposes, but I strongly suggest otherwise. Before you reach for your mortar and pestle, and grab a handful of your windowsill herbs, you first need to make sure that you know the basis of herbalism. One must develop a strong foundation to moderate one's expectations and returns.

## The Benefits of Herbalism

Herbalism involves the use of plants with therapeutic properties, from which the biological compounds are extracted and then used to treat various physical and mental health conditions. Herbal medicine is not some cryptic science without proven treatment methods. The World Health Organization (WHO) has estimated that approximately 80% of the overall population depends on natural medicine for some form of health care.

Apart from the obvious benefit of addressing health issues, there are many other reasons you should give herbalism a try:

<u>Economic Benefits</u> – One of the main reasons herbal medicine is so popular is because medicinal plants are quite cost-effective. You can summon up a large batch of remedies with just a few tablespoons of a single herb.

<u>Sense of Self-Reliance</u> – Knowing how to whip up your own natural medicaments means you are no longer dependent on the pharmaceutical industry for alleviating

every physical discomfort. There is a rewarding aspect to creating your own balms and potions. Whenever I take a glimpse at my well-stocked home apothecary, I feel a pleasant sense of accomplishment.

*Safe and Natural Alternative* – Creating your own herbal medicines means there is no guesswork involved, no wondering what is inside your remedy bottles. There are no hidden ingredients, and no harmful chemicals added. Think of it as squeezing nature's goodness straight into your jars.

*Healthier Alternative* – Herbal remedies really pack a punch. Unlike conventional medicine which is produced with the sole purpose of treating symptoms, medicinal plants go beyond addressing a certain health issue. Take rosemary, for instance. Rosemary infusion can act as a powerful remedy for treating migraines, but that's not the only thing it does. Rosemary is a decent source of vitamins A, $B_6$, and C, as well as the minerals calcium and iron. These medicaments are not only treating the ailment but giving you other benefits as well. This sure beats a chemical painkiller, doesn't it?

*It Gives You Options* – Herbs have different medicinal uses (more on those in the next section) that stimulate our cells. The best thing about making your homemade remedies is the ability to mix and match! You can combine herbs as you see fit, to address your unique conditions, and adjust their intensities in a way that works for your health. The possibilities are quite endless.

## The Anatomy of Herbs

It is easy to find out what medicinal effects a certain herb has on the body. Simple research can tell you which herbs you need to take for inflammation, calming your nerves, or alleviating pain. And that should work fine for a one-time remedy. But if you are serious about trying your hand at herbalism and creating plant-based medicaments, then you need a much deeper approach.

Apart from knowing the medicinal effects, you also need to understand the anatomy of herbs; different parts of the plants produce different compounds, all of which have certain actions within the body. Knowing a bit about the herbs' active constituents and their chemical compositions will help you understand how they work, which will kickstart your journey to becoming a master herbal healer.

**Volatile Oils** – Volatile oil is the plant's extract that we use for making essential oil. Usually composed of more than 100 different compounds, mostly monoterpenes (molecules with ten carbon atoms), it is one of the most important herbal constituents for medicinal purposes.

**Phenols** – Phenols are herbal constituents that are mainly antiseptic or anti-inflammatory in nature. They are usually produced by plants as a defense mechanism to protect themselves against external infection or grazing by insects. Some phenolic acids are powerful antioxidants and can even be antiviral. Phenols are a very varied group of organic compounds, but each compound is highly effective.

**Tannins** – Almost all plants produce tannins. Once again, this active constituent has the power to repel herbivorous insects. Tannin is a polyphenolic compound and a powerful astringent. In herbal medicine, this compound is mostly used for its ability to promote blood clotting and staunch bleeding. It also tightens relaxed tissues and is an effective cure for diarrhea and skin issues, such as eczema.

**Flavonoids** – Just like tannins, flavonoids are polyphenolic compounds that can be found in most plants. Flavonoids act as pigments, meaning they impart color (usually white or yellow) to fruits and flowers. This active constituent has many different medicinal effects, but the main reason we want to extract flavonoids is because of their powerful antioxidant uses. Plants that contain flavonoids are perfect for improving circulation, but they can also be used as anti-inflammatories, antivirals, and to protect the liver.

**Coumarins** – These active constituents can have quite different medicinal actions. Some plants containing coumarins stimulate the skin, while others can be powerful blood thinners and even muscle relaxants.

**Saponins** – If this word first reminds you of the word 'soap', you are not far from the truth. This active compound is called *saponin* because it makes a lather when it comes into contact with water, just like soap. Saponins can be expectorants (promote the secretion of mucus) and help with nutrient absorption, when in their *triterpenoid* form. When they occur in a *steroidal* form, these constituents have a powerful hormonal action.

**Alkaloids** – Pharmacologically speaking, alkaloids are active constituents due to their nitrogen-loaded chemical composition. Alkaloid plants help to create many popular conventional drugs, but they can have a powerful effect on the body, even in their raw, natural form. Alkaloid herbs can alleviate pain, reduce muscle spasms, and even help dry up secretions.

**Polysaccharides** – As the name suggests, polysaccharides contain sugar molecules. This constituent is found in all plants, but the most medicinally important ones are those that resemble a sticky gum, usually found in roots, bark, leaves, and seeds. These "gums" can soak up fluids, making them perfect for soothing and repairing irritated tissues or mucous membranes. Some polysaccharides also improve the immune system, for example, the sugar molecules found in aloe vera leaves.

**Bitters** – As you've already guessed, bitters are the active compounds in herbs that have a bitter or harsh taste. In theory, bitterness stimulates secretions in the digestive organs, so understandably, bitter medicinal plants can be perfect for improving and soothing digestive function. Bitters also allow the body to absorb nutrients more efficiently.

**Proanthocyanins** – Like flavonoids and tannins, proanthocyanins are also pigments, but these compounds give a darker hint of color – think blue, red, or purple flowers. This constituent is perfect for improving circulation in the heart, but also in the eyes, hands, and feet.

**Cyanogenic Glycosides** – As scary as the name sounds, cyanogenic glycosides can be quite helpful in tiny doses, despite producing toxic hydrogen cyanide when the plant is crushed. They act as a powerful relaxant that sedates the heart and muscles. In fact, the leaves, stems, seeds and roots of the elder tree contain these active substances, which is why their use can have a soothing effect.

**Cardiac Glycosides** – As the name suggests, these herbal constituents can protect the heart and entire cardiovascular system. They support the contraction rate and impact positively on the heart's function. But cardiac glycosides can also act as a diuretic and are incredibly helpful for urine production as well. Foxgloves are one of the best sources of these active compounds.

**Anthraquinones** – These herbal compounds do wonders for the large intestine. By causing contractions and stimulating the intestine walls, anthraquinones induce bowel movement and are a perfect natural laxative for treating irritating constipation.

**Glucosilinates** – This active constituent is only found in plants belonging to the cabbage and mustard family, and is often quite irritating for the skin, even causing blistering. However, when applied to joints as a poultice, these compounds can increase the blood flow and support healing.

**Minerals** – Just like all plants, medicinal herbs are packed with minerals. Many plants draw these beneficial compounds from the ground and then convert them into something easily broken down and absorbed by the body. For instance, dandelion leaves contain a high level of potassium, in addition to being a very powerful diuretic.

**Vitamins** – Although this is probably the most overlooked use for medicinal plants, many herbs have considerable vitamin content. In addition to their other therapeutic actions, herbs contain vitamins that increase their ability to heal your body. The more vitamins your body gets, the better your health will be.

## Speaking the Herbal Language

Before we get down to gathering herbs and extracting the active goodies trapped inside, it is beneficial to go through common terminology. Knowing the essential vocabulary and herbalism concepts will prepare you better to start this therapeutic practice on the right foot.

Whether we are discussing herbal actions, preparations, plant parts, or just common terms, this full herbal glossary is one that every aspiring herbalist should be familiar with:

<u>Abortifacient</u> – An action that induces abortion.

*Acetract/Acetum* – An herbal remedy that uses vinegar to extract the active compounds from herbs.

*Adaptogen* – Herbs that support the adrenal glands and help us adapt to and modulate physical and emotional stress.

*Adjuvant* – An agent which supports the actions of medicinal agents.

*Alterative* – An action that helps with chronic conditions because it removes metabolic wastes, boosts immunity, and cleanses the body.

*Amoebicidal* – Herbs that help with diseases caused by an amoeba.

*Amphoteric* – Actions that restore the normal functioning of organs.

*Anabolic* – Meaning to promote healthy tissue growth.

*Analeptic* – To stimulate and restore the normal functioning of the central nervous system.

*Analgesic* – An herbal action that relieves pain.

*Anaphrodisiac* – An action that is the opposite of aphrodisiac, meaning it reduces sexual desire and arousal.

*Anesthetic* – An action that induces anesthesia, numbness or loss of sensation by depressing certain nerve functions.

*Antacid* – An agent which neutralizes stomach acidity.

*Anti-anemic* – A medium which prevents anemia or helps with treating it, if already present.

*Antibacterial* – Prevents bacteria from spreading.

*Antibilious* – An action that combats stomachache, nausea, and other conditions that are caused by increased bile secretions.

*Antibiotic* – An action that inhibits bacterial growth.

*Anticancerous* – Prevents or decreases the risk of developing cancer.

*Anticatarrh* – Herbs that help with inflamed mucous membranes of throat and head.

*Antidepressant* – Medicinal action that prevents or decreases the intensity of mental depression.

*Antidiabetic* – An agent that helps with diabetes and may even improve the utilization of insulin.

*Antidiarrheal (antidiarrhetic)* – An action that prevents or treats diarrhea.

*Anti-emetic* – Alleviates and even prevents vomiting and nausea.

*Anti-epileptic* – An action that relieves symptoms of epilepsy and combats seizures.

*Antifungal* – An instrument used to destroy the growth of fungi.

*Antihemorrhagic* – Alleviates hemorrhaging and controls or prevents bleeding.

*Anti-infectious* – Stops or prevents infections.
*Anti-inflammatory* – An action that controls, reduces and prevents inflammation in the body.
*Antilithic* – Prevents kidney or bladder stones from forming.
*Antimalarial* – Relieves patient from symptoms or prevents malaria.
*Antimicrobial* – Herbs that destroy microbes.
*Antioxidant* – Prevents oxidation.
*Antiparasitic* – An action that prevents parasites from building up or treats parasitic conditions, if already present.
*Antiperiodic* – Herbal action that prevents diseases (like malaria) from reoccurring periodically.
*Antiphlogistic* – An action that counteracts inflammation.
*Antipruritic* – Prevents and relieves aggravating symptoms of itching.
*Antipyretic* – Reduces body fever and induces perspiration.
*Antirheumatic* – Prevents, treats, and eases the pain caused by rheumatism, an inflammation of the muscles and joints.
*Antiscorbutic* – Prevents and treats scurvy, a disease caused by vitamin C deficiency.
*Antiseptic* – An action that prevents decay, removes blood and pus, and inhibits the development of microorganisms.
*Antispasmodic* – Calms the nervous system and prevents and relieves muscle cramp and spasm.
*Antitussive* – Prevents, controls, and relieves coughing.
*Anti-ulcer* – Prevents ulcers from forming.
*Antivenomous* – An action that can act as a prevention to animal poison.
*Antiviral* – Works against viruses.
*Antizymotic* – An agent that prevents fermentation or decomposition.
*Anxiolytic* – Herbal action that prevents, relieves and reduces symptoms of anxiety.
*Aperient* – Works as a gentle laxative.
*Aperitive* – Herbs that are taken before meals to stimulate and increase appetite.
*Aphrodisiac* – Restores and increases sexual desire and arousal.
*Aromatherapy* – The art and practice of using essential oils to promote physical and emotional health. Aromatherapy stimulates the receptor sites in the brain, allowing the compounds from the oils to be absorbed.
*Aromatic* – Herbs that are rich in volatile oils and fragrant compounds.

*Asepsis* – Sterile and uninfected; free of germs.
*Astringent* – An action that causes the skin, blood vessels, and tissues to contract. It stops bleeding and mucus discharge.
*Aquaretic* – Increases urine production while retaining electrolytes. Great for improving blood circulation in the kidneys, but without affecting sodium resorption.
*Bactericidal* – Herbs that prevent bacterial infections.
*Balsam* – Soothing tree resin.
*Bronchial* – Improves respiration by relaxing spasms in the lungs and/or the tubes leading to them.
*Calmative* – Soothing actions with sedative properties.
*Carcinostatic* – Halting the growth of malignant tumors and carcinomas.
*Cardiotonic* – An action that strengthens the functioning of the heart.
*Carminative* – Prevents the formation of gas in the intestines and helps its release.
*Cathartic* – Induces bowel movement and causes evacuation. Cathartic herbs can be mild or vigorous.
*Caustic* – Herbs that are rich in acid that can cause corrosion on living tissues.
*Cephalic* – A term that refers to diseases on, in or near the head.
*Cholagogue* – An action that improves the flow of bile in the gallbladder.
*Cicatrizant* – Improves wound healing and supports the recovery of scar tissue.
*Cordial* – A stimulating herbal drink or medicine.
*Counterirritant* – An action that causes an inflammatory response of the affected area.
*Decongestant* – Relieves congestion.
*Demulcent* – Soothes, relieves, and protects irritated or inflamed mucous membrane, both internally and externally.
*Deobstruent* – Clears duct obstruction for the normal flow of secretions and bodily fluids.
*Depurative* – An action that purifies and cleanses the blood.
*Dermatitis* – Skin inflammation that results in itchiness and redness, also known as rash.
*Detergent* – Cleanses wounds, infections, ulcers, and boils.
*Diaphoretic* – An action that promotes perspiration and circulation, and eliminates surface toxins.
*Digestive* – Supports and promotes healthy digestion.
*Disinfectant* – Herbal action that destroys germs and pathogenic microbes that cause infections.

*Diuretic* – Herbal action that promotes the production and flow of urine.
*Ecbolic* – Increases uterine contractions.
*Emetic* – Herbs that induce and cause vomiting and the emptying of stomach contents.
*Emmenagogue* – Supports and regulates normal menstrual flow, but it can also clear blood congestion.
*Emollient* – Actions that soothe and soften the skin.
*Epispastic* – Substances that cause a discharge or blister to form.
*Errhine* – Herbal action that increases nasal secretion, as well as stimulating sneezing, when applied to the mucus membrane.
*Escharotic* – A substance that causes sloughing and kills tissue.
*Estrogenic* – An action that increases the production of the hormone estrogen, or acts as an estrogen.
*Euphoriant* – Sometimes addictive, this medicinal action causes the body to enter a temporary euphoric state.
*Exanthematous* – A remedy for measles, scarlet fever, and similar eruptive diseases of the skin.
*Exhilarant* – An herbal action that uplifts the mood and cheers the mind.
*Expectorant* – Supports the removal of the mucus from the trachea and lungs, although this term is often used to explain all sorts of remedies that can relieve coughs.
*Febrifuge* – An action that can decrease body temperature and fever. Very similar to antipyretic.
*Galactagogue* – Increases and supports the production and healthy flow of breast milk.
*Germicide* – An action that can destroy germs (pathogens).
*Hemagogue* – Supports and promotes healthy blood flow.
*Hemostatic* – Herbs that are astringent and can staunch or control bleeding, and purify the blood.
*Hepatic* – Increases bile secretion and promotes healthy liver function.
*Hypertensive* – An action that increases blood pressure.
*Hypnotic* – Relaxes the nervous system and supports sleep.
*Hypoglycemiant* – An action that lowers the blood sugar level.
*Hypotensive* – An action that lowers the blood pressure.
*Inhalation* – Breathing in steam through the nasal passage.
*Laxative* – Promotes the evacuation of bowel contents.
*Lithotriptic* – Substances that cause kidney and bladder stones to dissolve.
*Liniment* – An external remedy that is applied by rubbing.
*Masticatory* – Substances that increase the production of saliva

when chewing.
*Mucilage/Mucilaginous* – A sticky substance secreted by mucous membranes and glands.
*Mydriatic (also Myotic)* – An action that causes the pupils to dilate.
*Narcotic* – Addictive substance that reduces pain and induces drowsiness or sleep.
*Nauseant* – Causes vomiting and nausea.
*Nervine* – An action that relaxes the nervous system, soothes the nerves, and decreases tension.
*Nootropic* – Substances that improve cognitive functions and improve concentration and memory.
*Oxytocic* – An action that induces uterine contractions.
*Parasiticide* – Herbs that can destroy parasites.
*Parturifacient* – Induces labor and childbirth.
*Refrigerant* – Cooling actions that get rid of thirst and/or remove heat.
*Relaxant* – Substances that relax and get rid of anxiety and tension.
*Renal* – An action that strengthens, supports and treats kidney diseases and imbalances.
*Rubefacient* – Increases skin blood flow and induces redness.
*Sedative* – Substances that promote sleep and bring tranquility.
*Soporific* – Similar to a sedative. It promotes sleep.
*Spasmodic* – Causes muscle contraction and relaxation.
*Steroids* – Active organic compounds that include alkaloids, some vitamins and some hormones.
*Stimulant* – Stimulates and increases the functioning of a certain body part or organ, temporarily.
*Stomachic* – Promotes the health of the stomach and supports normal digestion.
*Terpenes* – Hydrocarbon molecules that are aromatic and form the base of volatile oils.
*Tonic* – Herbs that strengthen, restore, and nourish the entire body.
*Topical* – Form of remedy application that is used externally, on the body's surface.
*Thymoleptic* – Modifies mood and energizes mental health and wellbeing.
*Vermicide/Vermifuge* – Substance that destroys intestinal worms.
*Vulnerary* – Supports wound healing.

Now that you know how medicinal plants work and why you should give herbalism a try, the real fun can begin. Let's dive deeper into the therapeutic side of nature, so that we can learn how to allow it to heal us from the inside out.

# The Most Effective Herbs to Know, Grow and Use

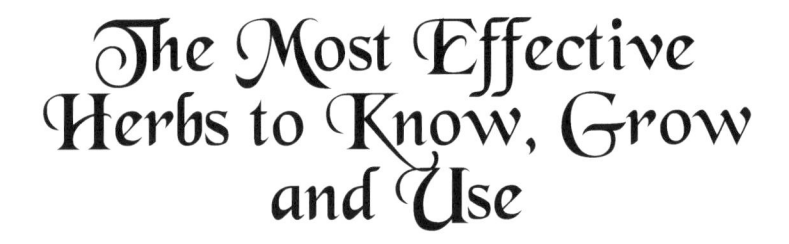

Herbs are the cornerstone of healing, and they have been used for medicinal practices for thousands of years. They may be masked by various chemical processes, but plant compounds still form the foundation of many pharmaceuticals that we use today. Did you know that aspirin is derived from willow bark? No, I am not railing against the use of modern drugs; I am simply trying to emphasize the potency that natural herbs have. When your body starts to shoot off painful signals, it is tempting to reach for that bottle of pills – but there is an alternative!

Herbs comprise many active components, each bringing something new and different to the body. They produce various chemical compounds that can protect against, or help treat, many diseases and illnesses. Depending on what health concerns you are looking to address, there are many herbs, or parts of plants, that you can use to your advantage.

To break free from the unnecessary shackles of the pharmaceutical industry, I present to you the 40 essential herbs that will help you build your natural apothecary at home.

## Your Natural First-Aid Kit

We all have a first-aid kit somewhere around the house, in the trunk of our car, or stashed somewhere else; while this conventional suitcase is well-equipped to assist us when we are in an accident, that doesn't mean that we should reach for chemically-loaded creams for every scrape. Enriching the medical bag with natural supplements not only gives you more options to choose from when a sudden injury strikes, but also helps you limit the use of pharmaceuticals when it is not necessary.

To make sure you are shielded from all sorts of misfortunes, here are the top 12 herbs that every green healer wannabe should never run out of.

## ARNICA
### *(Arnica montana)*

Arnica montana is a powerful homeopathic that is mostly used for relieving muscle pain. A 2007 study found that arnica gel was just as effective as Ibuprofen gel when given to patients with finger osteoarthritis (Widrig et al., 2007). Both groups had a similar recovery, and the doctors had a difficult time distinguishing between those patients who received the arnica, and those who received the Ibuprofen gel.

My husband often has claudication (leg cramps when walking) so, whenever we take our long walks or go hiking, I always have my arnica gel with me. I remember once he started experiencing severe calf pain, and he could barely move. We sat on the ground, and I massaged this amazing gel into the skin on his leg for about ten minutes or so. Half an hour later, he was ready to race me to the top of the hill.

**Native to:** Europe, Northwestern US, Canada, the Pyrenees Mountains, Siberia

**Description:** When harvested in full bloom, arnica is recognizable by its yellow flowers and egg-shaped leaves. Arnica is mostly used as a natural ointment and compression for sprains and bruises. It kickstarts the healing process and relieves muscle pain. It can be used, internally, for treating shock or injury, but this is a rare application and requires dilution. The plant can be quite toxic (even if the dose is low), so internal consumption is <u>not recommended.</u>

Arnica cream or gel can be the perfect addition to your natural first-aid kit and effective for healing bruises or decreasing muscle aches.

**Main Components:** Flavonoids, sesquiterpene lactones, volatile oil, polysaccharides, mucilage, thymol

**Medicinal Actions:**
Homeopathic
Anti-inflammatory

**Main Uses:**
Relieves Muscle Pain
Heals Bruises and Sprains
Improves Blood Supply Locally
Reabsorbs Internal Bleeding

**Parts Used:** The flowers and rhizome

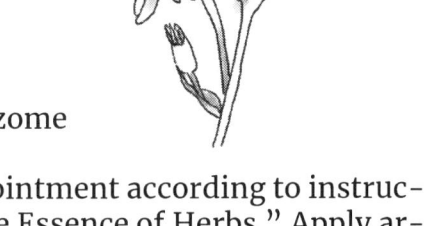

**Practical use:** Compression and ointment according to instructions in the chapter "Harnessing the Essence of Herbs." Apply arnica for anti-inflammation effects. It works wonders!

**Safety Precautions:** Arnica, in its pure form, can be quite poisonous when taken internally. Use only for external application and only when the skin is healthy. Applying arnica on broken skin can cause dermatitis.

## CALENDULA
*(Calendula officinalis)*

Calendula tinctures are probably the most effective natural tissue-repairing and redness-soothing remedy. Its pharmacological properties and high anti-inflammatory constituents make calendula the safest wash for infants' diaper rash.

I always keep a calendula ointment in my first-aid kit bag, as it always comes in handy in late spring, when the sun gets a bit too hot for my skin. The herb also makes fantastic natural gargles for sore throats and blisters. A few years back, when I was going through a tough period, doctors diagnosed that stress was causing painful blisters in my mouth. If it hadn't been for my calendula gargles to relieve these sores, I would probably have been even more stressed.

**Native to:** Southern Europe

**Description:** You may know it as pot marigold, that lovely orange flower sitting decoratively in your garden. But what you may not be aware of is that calendula is packed with medicinal properties that should grant it a place in your first-aid kit. Primarily used as a remedy for the skin, calendula can soothe inflamed skin, rashes, and sunburns, and is also effective for cuts and scrapes. When taken internally, these bright orange petals support digestion and help against gut inflammation issues.

**Main Components:** Flavonoids, resins, phytosterols, carotenes, bitter glycosides, mucilage, volatile oil.

**Medicinal Actions:**
Anti-inflammatory
Antiviral
Antibacterial
Detoxifying
Heals Wounds
Relieves Muscle Spasms
Mildly Estrogenic

**Main Uses:**
Soothes Red and Inflamed Skin (rashes, burns, acne)
Treats Fungal Conditions (thrush, athlete's foot, ringworm)
Treats *Candida albicans* Efficiently
Heals Cuts and Wounds (it astringes the capillaries)
Supports Digestion
Helps with Ulcers and Gastritis
Gynecological Uses

**Parts Used:** The flowers: the petals and the flower head

**Practical use:** Suitable for making infusions, infused oils, creams, ointments, and tinctures.

**Safety Precautions:** Don't take calendula internally during pregnancy. It can also cause drowsiness if combined with post-surgery medications, and chronic sleepiness if consumed with sedatives.

# COMFREY
### (Symphytum officinale)

Comfrey is one of the most powerful natural healers. My homemade ointment is always in my medical kit to assist with sprains and bruises. Accompanying my husband on his hiking adventures goes against my clumsy nature, as I always seem to find a huge rock on which to sprain my ankle. My record was last fall when my clumsiness clashed with rainy weather and a slippery path. I seemed always to be injuring myself. Multiple times on the trail, I twisted my ankle. I thought my husband would have to carry me all the way back but, after 20 minutes of rubbing the ointment on my injury, I was actually able to get up and walk normally. Comfrey may not be magical, but it sure is effective.

*Don't just blindly believe me. Research from the* Complementary Therapies in Medicine *(Frost et al., 2013) suggests that comfrey is quite effective in healing abrasive wounds.*

**Native to:** Europe

**Description:** If you live in a temperate region, you have probably come across comfrey before. With thick leaves and a cluster of (usually) pink flowers, this shrub grows throughout the world. Comfrey, literally meaning *made firm*, has a long history of traditional use for mending bones. In fact, the common names for comfrey are knitbone and boneset, because of this classic application. It can also be used for healing wounds and ruptures. Today, this beneficial plant is a popular natural supplement used to treat sports injuries, thanks to its powerful ability to support the healing of bruises, fractures, and sprains. Comfrey can also be used for treating insect bites or other skin-inflammation issues.

**Main Components:** Mucilage, phenolic acids, allantoin, asparagine, triterpenoids, tannins

**Medicinal Actions:**
Anti-inflammatory
Demulcent

Tissue-repairing Properties
Wound-healing Actions
Astringent

**Main Uses:**
Supports the Healing of Bruises
Knits Together Ligaments and Bones
Reduces the Severity of Sprains as Compress
Applied for Graze Soothing
Heals Insects Bites
Used for Treating Mastitis

**Parts Used:** Entire plant – roots and aerial parts

**Practical use:** Feel free to make a compress, tincture, ointment or infused oil out of comfrey, for the desired outcome.

**Safety Precautions:** Comfrey can be unsafe for internal use as it has been linked to liver damage. For this reason, it has become a much-maligned plant. It is certainly one herb that should be used under the guidance of a practitioner until you have sufficient experience of your own. It is very valuable for use internally, and in the short term, once you know how to use it. When applying externally, make sure that the skin is healthy and not broken, as the chemicals in comfrey can cause further damage.

## ECHINACEA
*(Echinacea spp.)*

Scientists have concluded that consuming echinacea might knock down the risk of catching a cold by 58% (Shah et al., 2007). If you are already fighting a cold, the same scientists found out that taking echinacea can shorten the time you spend in bed by 1.4 days.

Last winter, I was on a weekend trip to the Alps, and the whole family got a cold in the middle of our ski trip. We had paid for everything in advance and were really looking forward to having some fun. You could only imagine how annoyed we were about having to spend the rest of our trip in bed. Since I'd brought my herbal kit along, I thought it would be a good idea for us to take an echinacea pill before going to bed. And boy, was I right. The next day, our cold symptoms were almost gone, and we had a memorable time out in the snow.

**Native to:** Central USA

**Description:** Previously referred to as *snakeroot*, echinacea is a purple daisy-like perennial packed with infection-fighting and toxin-cleansing properties. Traditionally used as a cure for snake bites, sore throat, and septic issues, this coneflower can be a powerful natural remedy for viral and bacterial conditions. Although echinacea's medicinal history is not a very long list, today, snakeroot is one of the most commonly used plants in Western herbal medicine. Echinacea can be used for various diseases, especially those related to infection.

**Main Components:** Polysaccharides, caffeic acid esters, alkylamines

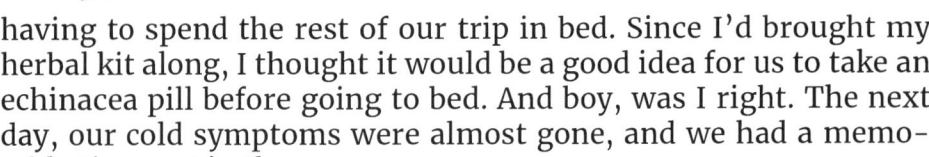

**Medicinal Actions:**
Detoxifying
Anti-inflammatory
Wound Healing Properties
Antimicrobial
Immune Modulating
Increases White Blood Cell Count

**Main Uses:**
Remedy for Infections
Relieves Sore Throats
Relieves Acne and Other Skin Infections
Treats Asthma and Similar Allergies
Flu and Cold Remedy
Relieves Skin from Bites and Stings

**Parts Used:** The flower and root

**Practical use:** Echinacea is awesome as a tincture, when made into capsules or tablets, or a decoction.

**Safety Precautions:** Echinacea is generally safe for both internal and external use. However, keep in mind that echinacea interacts with caffeine. Taking echinacea with coffee will slow the breakdown of caffeine, and you may end up with too much caffeine in the bloodstream.

# FEVERFEW
*(Tanacetum parthenium)*

Research says that feverfew has the potential to be considered the natural drug for treating migraines (Pittler & Ernst, 2004). It reduces the frequency and severity of migraines but is not for aspirin-like pain relief of other types of headaches. It has anti-inflammatory properties and is believed to increase the release of serotonin and decrease the release of histamines. Instead of reaching for a painkiller, why not try to soothe the ache the herbal way. The extract of this herb, in the form of capsules, is my go-to for reducing the severity of migraines.

A few months back, I was headed to a conference in another country, with my husband. I always have a mean headache after a long drive, and this time was no different. Just as I thought that I would spend the whole day in agony, I popped one of my feverfew capsules, and 2 hours later, the symptoms of my migraine were gone. Surprisingly enough, my head didn't hurt on our trip back home either.

**Native to:** Southeastern Europe

**Description:** At first glance, you might confuse this plant with chamomile. Despite both belonging to the Chrysanthemum family, and sharing the same white, daisy-like flower with a yellow center, these two plants are different. Unlike chamomile, it is the leaves of the feverfew that are packed with therapeutic properties. Traditionally referred to as "the woman's herb," feverfew has been used for inducing menstruation for many centuries. Now mainly used for treating migraines, feverfew is a must-have among your herbal supplements. Keep it in your first-aid kit for quick relief.

**Main Components:** Volatile oil, sesquiterpenes, sesquiterpene lactones

**Medicinal Actions:**
Analgesic
Anti-inflammatory
Antirheumatic
Supports the Menstrual Cycle
Reduces Fevers

**Main Uses:**
Lowers Body Temperature
Induces Menstruation
Prevents Migraine
Decreases Arthritic and Rheumatic Pain

**Parts Used:** The aerial parts (the parts that grow above ground)

**Practical use:** Go right ahead and make a tincture, capsules or tablets, or just use the fresh leaves for consumption. So easy! It can't get any better than that!

**Safety Precautions:** Avoid chewing fresh leaves and internal consumption during pregnancy. Feverfew is also known to impair blood clotting, so avoid using before and after surgery.

## GARLIC
*(Allium sativum)*

Garlic can be a powerful antibiotic, which is great for treating infections. Scientists have found that, under certain circumstances, its compound diallyl sulfide is a whopping 100 times more effective than other conventional antibiotics used for slaying the Campylobacter bacterium, the main culprit for gut infections (Lu et al., 2012). You may not be a big fan of your garlic breath, but your health will surely appreciate your consumption of the plant.

When visiting Chicago last year, my daughter started experiencing terrible pain in her ear. She always has trouble with the nerves around the ear canals when the temperature drops and she doesn't have her hat on. Just as she started to complain, I gave her a garlic capsule (an extract I always keep in my first-aid kit). After

30 to 40 minutes, when I asked her if she was feeling better, she smiled, surprised, and said, "Oh, I already forgot about the pain. I guess your magical pills do work!"

**Native to:** Central Asia

**Description:** If your grandma used to chew on garlic cloves to knock down her blood pressure, you already know of the amazing benefits of this pungent bulbous perennial. Garlic does not only enhance our meals, but it also improves our health. It fights infections, keeps our blood pressure, cholesterol, and blood sugar in check, and it is one of the most popular natural supplements. Experts say the best way to squeeze out the healthy antimicrobial compounds from garlic is to crush, dice or otherwise break the cloves to allow conversion of chemicals to allicin, and other antibiotic goodies, before tincturing or eating. Wait 10 minutes after crushing, and then use this as a medicine or ingest with food. Garlic's well-known odor comes from the sulfur compounds that it contains.

Garlic extract, in the form of capsules, can be the perfect addition to your first-aid bag to take care of sudden infections.

**Main Components:** Volatile oil, selenium, scordinin, vitamin A, B, C, E, allicin

**Medicinal Actions:**
Antibiotic
Antidiabetic
Anti-inflammatory
Expectorant
Blood Pressure Regulator
Sweat Inducer

**Main Uses:**
Lowers High Blood Pressure
Aid for Type 2 Diabetes
Treats Infections (mostly for the throat, nose, chest, ears)
Prevents and Breaks Down Blood Clots
Helps Treat Fungal Skin Conditions
Protects from Cancers, Such as Stomach and Colon Cancers

**Parts Used:** The whole plant (mostly the bulb)

**Practical use:** Suitable for raw consumption, syrups, capsules or tablets. All work wonderfully, depending on your needs.

**Safety Precautions:** Garlic is known to lower blood sugar and blood pressure, so use with caution if you already have low blood pressure or sugar, as the levels may drop too low for you. Also, raw garlic, applied to the skin, may cause irritations in some cases.

## LAVENDER
*(Lavandula spp.)*

In the 17th century, the herbalist John Parkinson wrote about lavender, saying it was "good for the griefs and pains of the head and brain." I'm here in the 21st century to confirm what Parkinson said. A 2014 study found that consuming lavender essential oil treated anxiety more effectively than a tranquilizer (Chevallier, 2016, p. 108). But this lovely-scented herb is more than just a relaxant. Its essential oil is great for treating insect bites and burns, making it a great addition to a natural first-aid kit.

A couple of years back, we went camping with some friends. I went with my daughter a day earlier, and my husband was supposed to join us the next day. I had forgotten my herbal kit, so I asked him to bring it along. The first night we endured so many mosquito bites that we spent the next day scratching our skin off. Once he brought my lavender oil, we applied it onto the affected areas, and the irritation started to wear off. My husband also treated his own skin as a preventative measure. Take a guess as to how many mosquito bites he endured that evening . . . None!

**Native to:** Western Mediterranean, especially France

**Description:** Lavender can do more than just soothe you during a relaxing soak in the bath. You may primarily know it to be a scent in your cosmetic products or room fresheners, but lavender has powerful medicinal properties as well. When used internally, the purple flowers can be a great antidepressant, while external applications work as an insecticide. And thanks to the high content of volatile oil, lavender will also keep the health of your gut in check.

Lavender essential oil has proven to be an invaluable remedy that can even relieve headaches, if gently massaged on the temples.

**Main Components:** Volatile oil, flavonoids

**Medicinal Actions:**
Antidepressant
Antispasmodic
Neuroprotective
Antimicrobial

**Main Uses:**
Relaxant for Reducing Stress and Anxiety
Sedative Effect
Soothes Indigestion
Soothes Insect Bites
Antiseptic for Burns, Wounds and Sores

**Parts Used:** The flowers

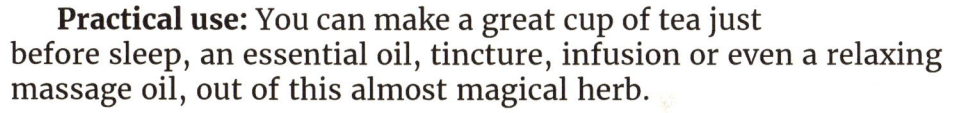

**Practical use:** You can make a great cup of tea just before sleep, an essential oil, tincture, infusion or even a relaxing massage oil, out of this almost magical herb.

**Safety Precautions:** When applying the essential oil topically, make sure to use small, medicinal amounts, as lavender can sometimes cause irritation if the dosage is higher. Also, avoid taking lavender with sedatives, as it might cause chronic sleepiness. Lavender oil is also estrogenic, so avoid using large amounts over long periods of time; for this reason, lavender oil can cause problems for children, especially small boys.

## MYRRH
*(Commiphora molmol)*

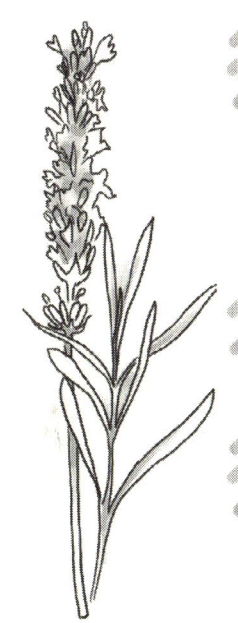

Known as "the Wise Man's Cure," myrrh was one of the gifts that baby Jesus received from the Three Wise Men. Known as one of the oldest medicinal herbs, ancient Egyptians depended on this beneficial tree for treating herpes and hay fever. Today, studies have found that myrrh helps with neuropathic pain and rheumatoid arthritis (Chevallier, 2016, p. 85), and is a key weapon against many infections. In fact, it is one of the most powerful weapons we will discuss. One study found that myrrh extract clears liver fluke infections in a matter of weeks (Massoud et al., 2001).

And I can attest to that! Three years ago, I started experiencing severe diarrhea and abdominal pain. I went to my doctor, and he told me it was caused by liver fluke. I researched and found out that myrrh – my sore-throat remedy – was perfect for it. In a couple of days, I wasn't feeling any more symptoms. A week after that, on my next checkup, my doctor was surprised at how I had cleansed myself with nothing but herbs. Like a green doctor in the forest, you too can mix up your own powders and potions to become more powerful.

**Native to:** Northeast Africa

**Description:** You may know myrrh as the distinct scent used in conventional mouthwashes, but in its natural state, this gummy resin oozes out of the cuts of the myrrh tree's bark. When dried, myrrh turns yellow-red, resembling raisins. Packed with anti-inflammatory properties, and having a rich, bitter taste, this gum is quite beneficial for relieving coughs, asthma, and sore throats, which is why it deserves a spot in your first-aid kit.

**Main Components:** Gum, volatile oil, resin

**Medicinal Actions:**
Anti-inflammatory
Anticancerous
Antiseptic
Antiparasitic
Anti-ulcer
Astringent

**Main Uses:**
Clears the Body of Parasitic Infections, Especially Liver Fluke
   A Remedy for the Mouth and Throat
   Ayurvedic Remedy and Tonic
   Cures Ulcers
   Relieves Congestion

Clears Oral Thrush
Treats Acne and other Skin Problems

**Parts Used:** The gum (resin)

**Practical use:** Myrrh can be used in tinctures, mouthwashes, powders, capsules and essential oils.

**Safety Precautions:** Follow the instructions for the dosage well, before consuming, as large doses of myrrh can cause kidney irritation and changes in the heart rate. Also, myrrh interacts with blood sugar medications, so avoid using this herb if you are already taking drugs for diabetes.

## TEA TREE
*(Melaleuca alternifolia)*

It was Captain James Cook who introduced this Aboriginal remedy to the Western world in the 1770s. He had sipped a tea made from the leaves of this species of tea tree, to prevent scurvy, and asked the Aborigines (indigenous Australian people) to share its healing secrets with him. When he brought tea tree oil back to the west for the doctors to test its powers, it was confirmed that tea tree oil was a better antiseptic than the then popular aloe vera. Tea tree oil was extensively used before the discovery of penicillin. In fact, in WW2, wounded Australian soldiers were given tea tree oil to prevent infections.

My friend, who has the most sensitive skin, got athlete's foot on her last vacation. She said she had spent her days in the hotel's swimming pool – a breeding ground for the fungus. She called me the minute she noticed it, to ask what she should put on her fungal infection. I told her to use tea tree oil, which she found in a local health store. Three days after that, she sent me a picture of her freshly pedicured feet without any sign of the ugly infection.

**Native to:** Australia

**Description:** The pointed leaves of the tea tree, and especially their essential oil, are the most effective antiseptic found in nature. First officially confirmed as effective in Australia in 1923, tea tree is a traditional Aboriginal remedy that has been intensively researched since the sixties. The leaves can be crushed and inhaled for coughs, or used as infusions for skin problems. Tea tree has been an effective healer of many infections: skin, oral, gynecological, and even chronic.

**Main Components:** Volatile oil

**Medicinal Actions:**
Antiseptic
Antifungal
Antibacterial
Antiviral
Immune Stimulant

**Main Uses:**
Treats Cystitis
Treats Skin Infections (ringworm, athlete's foot)
Relieves Boils and Acne
Treats Vaginal Infections
Treats Gum Disease
Sore Throat Gargle
Relieves Coughs
Helps Treat Chronic Fatigue Syndrome

**Parts Used:** The leaves

**Practical use:** Good for making essential oils, infusions, and creams.

**Safety Precautions:** Do not consume tea tree internally. Also, don't apply tea tree oil topically if it is undiluted, as it can cause irritation.

## THYME
*(Thymus vulgaris)*

Thymol is a powerful volatile oil found in thyme. This chemical compound plays an important part in hand sanitizers, mouthwashes, and acne meditation today. In the 19th century, Victorian nurses used to soak their bandages in thyme-diluted water to stop infections from spreading. Before the modern era of refrigerators, monasteries depended on thyme to store their food without it spoiling.

A few winters back, the weather was deceptively warm. I was out Christmas shopping a few days in advance, so I thought leaving my coat in the car would be a good idea. When sweaty skin and low temperatures mix, chest infection is almost guaranteed. My thyme syrup helped me power through the coughs and the infection. By the time Christmas rolled around, I was sipping on champagne.

**Native to:** Southern Europe

**Description:** Thyme is more than just the herb you use to spice up your pork chops or roast chicken. It is the superstar of your windowsill garden, not only because of its uncanny ability to make holiday food delicious – though that is undeniable – but also because of its powerful medicinal properties. For centuries, it has been used as a cough remedy; and when used to make syrup, it can battle serious respiratory issues. It is also great for infections and as an immune-boosting tonic.

**Main Components:** Volatile oil

**Medicinal Actions:**
Antiseptic
Expectorant
Tonic
Antioxidant
Antispasmodic

**Main Uses:**
Treats Asthma Symptoms
Relieves Coughs and Respiratory Issues
Effective in Dealing with Chest Infections
Tonic for the Immune System
Helps Expel Worms
Relieves Bites and Stings

**Parts Used:** The aerial parts (that grow above ground)

**Practical use:** Another great herb for making an essential oil, syrup, infusion, or tincture.

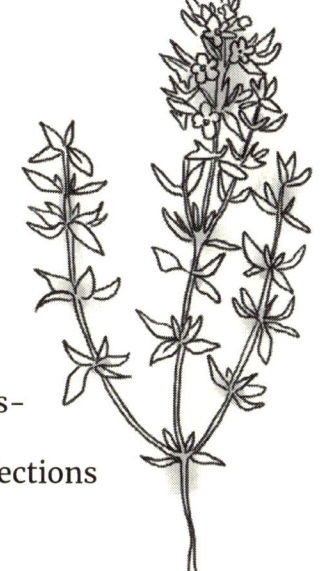

**Safety Precautions:** Thyme can slow down blood clotting and may increase bleeding, so be wary of how you use this herb if undergoing a surgery. Taking thyme with anticoagulant medications is not recommended.

# VALERIAN
*(Valeriana officinalis)*

Derived from the Latin "valere" which translates as "to be well," valerian is one of the most powerful herbs around. This is an herb that knocks down stress, aids sleep, and soothes the being. In war-torn Sarajevo (Bosnia and Herzegovina), back in 1993, doctors depended on Valeriana officinalis to treat traumatized soldiers. This was at a time when medical supplies were unavailable. Valerian has been a popular relaxant since Roman times, and studies have found it to be as effective as sedative drugs such as oxazepam.

Our friends have a beautiful five-year-old boy. When he was three and a half years old, they moved to a new apartment, and he started experiencing trouble falling asleep. He would wake up after ten minutes and cry for an hour. His pediatrician had prescribed a medication, but it wasn't helpful. I suggested an herbal valerian supplement. Three days after that, they called to thank me for restoring their beauty sleep again.

**Native to:** Europe, Northern Asia

**Description:** Thanks to its non-addictive and relaxing properties, valerian has become one of the safest and most effective sedatives in the world. Its rhizome and root are also used for treating epilepsy because they decrease mental over-activity. It is recommended to those people who cannot "switch off" because it has a powerful calming effect. It is the perfect addition to your first-aid kit for when you need a booster to bring back the feel-good vibes. When combined with other herbs, valerian can also help lower blood pressure.

**Main Components:** Volatile oil, alkaloids, iridoids

**Medicinal Actions:**
Relaxant
Sedative

Antispasmodic
Anxiety Relief

**Main Uses:**
Improves Sleep
Relieves Stress
Relieves Anxiety
Relieves Panic and Tremor
Reduces Sweating
Relaxes Contracting Muscles
Helps with Neck and Shoulder Tension

**Parts Used:** The root and rhizome

**Practical use:** Prepare this amazing herb as a tincture, tablets, decoction, or a powder to extract the benefits.

**Safety Precautions:** Generally safe for both internal and external use. However, valerian slows down the central nervous system, so it can be harmful if taken with anesthetics or before and after surgery. It can also do the reverse, and act as a stimulant in a small percentage of the population, particularly the clinically hyperactive.

## WITCH HAZEL
*(Hamamelis virginiana)*

Originally called "The Golden Treasure," witch hazel was the first mass-marketed herbal remedy in America. It was developed in 1846 by an American pharmacist (T. T. Pond), and marketed as Pond's Extract (Gartrell, 2000). Despite its name, witch hazel has nothing to do with the occult or with stirring up potions. It originates from the Middle English "wicke" which means "lively" or "bendable." Wicke is a word used to describe the Y-shaped stick used in the ancient technique of searching for underground water. But even if it does not refer to witches, that doesn't mean it lacks magical prowess. When it comes to soothing irritated skin, cleaning wounds, and reducing inflammation, this plant has been found, in studies, to be an effective treatment (Wolff & Kieser, 2007).

A small bottle with distilled witch hazel water is always in my first-aid kit. When we were visiting France's countryside, I fell off my bike and hurt my knee quite badly. I told you I was clumsy! The injury was so bad that I needed stitches. I cleaned my knee with my witch hazel water that was in the kit in my backpack. When I finally got to the hospital, three hours later, the nurse told me that she had never seen anyone do such a good job at cleaning a wound before. I told her it was nothing but some witch hazel, and she was quite impressed with my herbal knowledge.

**Native to:** Canada, Eastern USA

**Description:** Yellow flowers that bloom in the freezing winter? This may have been the first hint to the Native North Americans that there was something mysterious about this plant. Whatever force persuaded them to try the mystical plant, we surely must thank it. The Food and Drug Administration approves witch hazel as a natural non-prescription drug. A powerful remedy for inflammations, wound cleaning, skin issues, and insect stings, this plant is versatile enough to bring benefits to several elements of your life.

**Main Components:** Tannins, volatile oil (the leaves only), flavonoids, bitters

**Medicinal Actions:**
Anti-inflammatory
Astringent
Stops Bleeding (internal and external)

**Main Uses:**
Protects and Heals Broken Skin
Cleans Wounds
Treats Eczema
Repairs Damaged Facial Veins
Tightens Distended Veins
Eyewash for Eye Inflammation
Treats Diarrhea
Reduces Heavy Menstrual Flow
Soothes Insect Bites

**Parts Used:** The leaves and bark

**Practical use:** This is an old favorite of mine and you can prepare it as a tincture, distilled witch hazel, infusion, and as an ointment.

**Safety Precautions:** Though generally safe for everyone, a special precaution should be taken with dosages, as large amounts of witch hazel, consumed internally, may cause liver issues.

These 12 herbs cover a wide range of medicinal uses and form the ultimate natural first-aid kit. Unless you absolutely need to choose a conventional aggressive medication (sometimes garlic will not do the trick, and you will need a pharmaceutical antibiotic), I suggest you pack the herbal remedies into your handy medicine bag and keep this bag with you at all times.

## Other Essential Herbs for the Home Apothecary

Apart from the plants that can practice first aid, many other herbs are also full of medicinal properties for your overall health. From agrimony to yarrow, here are the essential herbs that you should understand and master if you want to practice your herbal healing skills. For centuries, all these herbs and plants have been pressed, steeped, or infused to aid in the healing of the human body.

### AGRIMONY
*(Agrimonia eupatoria)*

We have come a long way since placing agrimony sprigs under the bed for a good night's sleep, as British folklore dictates. We've also improved since the Anglo-Saxonian way of boiling agrimony in milk for erectile purposes. As Michael Drayton, an English poet who lived from 1563–1631, said, "agrimony is really an 'all-heal'." Many studies later, we think the same way! From staunching bleeding to being used as a tonic to aid digestion, this versatile plant can support our health in many different ways.

Whenever my daughter has diarrhea, I prepare agrimony tea and give it to her twice a day. The next day, the symptoms are almost gone, and her digestion is much improved

**Native to:** Europe

**Description:** Herbalists dry the aerial parts and the seeds of this mildly aromatic plant. Agrimony has a long history as a wound healer, thanks to its clot-forming properties, but it is also widely used as a tonic for treating diarrhea and supporting digestion. In Traditional Chinese Medicine, agrimony is the go-to herb for stopping bleeding and heavy menstruation.

When combined with other herbs, it can also treat urinary tract and kidney conditions.

**Main Components:** Flavonoids, coumarins, polysaccharides, bitters, tannins, vitamins B and K

**Medicinal Actions:**
Anti-inflammatory
Diuretic
Astringent
Tonic
Cholagogue
Hemostatic

**Main Uses:**
Heals Wounds
Coagulates Blood
Relieves Diarrhea
Increases Blood Flood
Supports Digestion
Liver Tonic
Helpful for Rashes and Acne

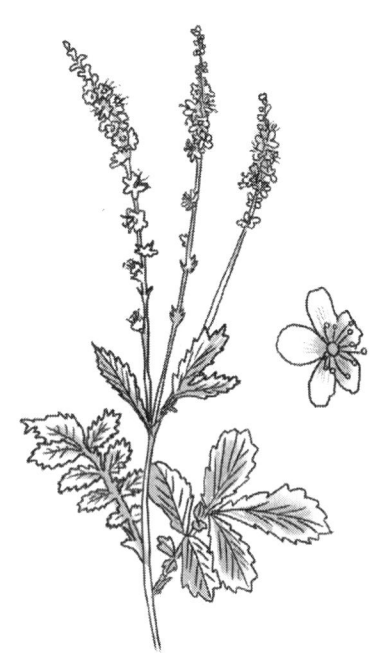

**Parts Used:** The parts that grow above the ground (stems, leaves, flowers)

**Practical use:** The tea is probably the fastest and easiest to make but you can also prepare a tincture, compresses, and eye baths to treat discharge and inflammation.

**Safety Precautions:** Avoid agrimony during pregnancy and breastfeeding. Do not consume more than 3 g a day, internally. Agrimony lowers blood sugar levels, so avoid taking agrimony with medications for diabetes.

# ALOE VERA
*(Aloe barbadensis)*

Aloe vera is one of the oldest medicinal herbs on this planet. As legends report, the ancient Greek philosopher, Aristotle, advised Alexander the Great, a powerful ruler of Macedonia, to conquer an African island to stock up on aloe vera supplies. This would allegedly cure his wounded soldiers. More than 2200 years later, Japanese soldiers in WW2 also used this plant's gel to heal their wounds in a natural way. Aloe vera may be an old-time plant, but it surely gives us a timeless cure!

Last Christmas, I was so busy in the kitchen preparing supper I burned my hand quite badly on the stove. When my husband saw the burn, he was concerned for me and thought that it would leave a huge scar. I treated my hand with aloe vera gel for a few days, and voila! The mark faded rapidly and disappeared into the mist, never to be seen again.

**Native to:** North Africa, Southern Europe

**Description:** Aloe vera is extensively cultivated as a potted plant worldwide, and it is one of the most commonly used plants for beauty and skin treatments. Cleopatra, the ruler of Egypt from 52–31 BC, the real-life Aphrodite, attributed her timeless beauty to aloe. So, it is clear that aloe was being used a very long time ago. Aloe vera has two main medicinal uses: a gel from the leaves that is used for healing wounds and treating burns; and the dried, powdered, yellow sap from the leaves, used as a bitter laxative for constipation. Herbalists cut the leaves open to scrape the gel, and then they drain them to collect the bitter liquid.

**Main Components:** Anthraquinones, tannins, resins, Aloectin B, polysaccharides

**Medicinal Actions:**
Heals
Laxative
Emollient
Stimulates Bile Secretion

**Main Uses:**

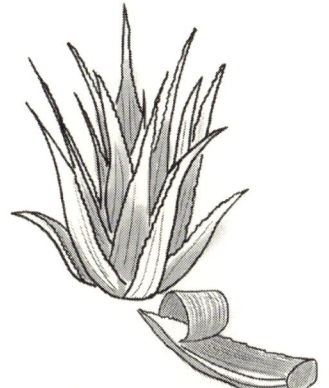

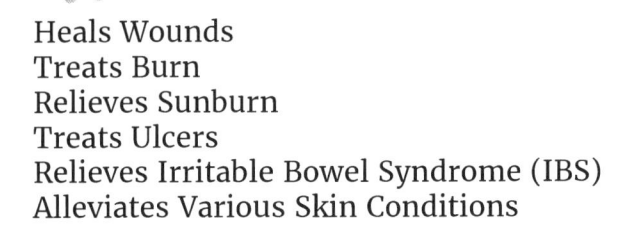

Heals Wounds
Treats Burn
Relieves Sunburn
Treats Ulcers
Relieves Irritable Bowel Syndrome (IBS)
Alleviates Various Skin Conditions

**Parts Used:** The leaves, broken for the gel and drained for the liquid

**Practical use:** Make the famous aloe gel, juice, or tincture to extract the medicines you desire.

**Safety Precautions:** People who are allergic to garlic and onion may also be allergic to aloe vera. Do not apply to severe burns and deep cuts, as it may have an adverse effect.

## ANGELICA
*(Angelica officinalis)*

With over 4000 years of use in Traditional Chinese Medicine, Angelica is one of the oldest medicinal herbs popular among natural-healing practitioners worldwide. The name is derived from a 17th-century monk's dream in which St. Michael told him to use this plant to cure the bubonic plague. It was considered an "angel" on earth and chronicles report that people at that time believed that chewing angelica root all day would make them immune to the plague.

One of my closest friends began struggling with her menstrual cycle after giving birth. She tried all sorts of hormonal medications prescribed by her gynecologist, but nothing did the trick. I recommended she give an angelica infusion a shot. After a couple of weeks, everything went back to functioning normally.

**Native to:** The Northern Hemisphere (subarctic and temperate regions)

**Description:** The genus Angelica contains about 60 different species with Norwegian, American, and Chinese angelica being the most popular ones. Angelica is a tall plant with bipinnate leaves and green or whiteish flowers grouped together into large umbels. Used for medicinal properties, angelica is a powerful natural tonic that treats many conditions specific to women, as well as heartburn, anemia, intestinal gas, and circulation. It is also used to treat hair loss because it causes increased circulation in the scalp. In China, dong quai angelica (*Angelica sinensis*) is mainly used for its property of causing uterine contractions and as a natural gynecological supplement.

**Main Components:** Volatile oils, ferulic acid, coumarins, polyacetylenes, phytosterols

**Medicinal Actions:**
Antispasmodic
Anti-inflammatory
Blood Thinner

Tonic
Stomachic

**Main Uses:**
Helps Uterine Contraction
Supports Healthy Menstrual Flow
Used for Treating Anemia, or Other Blood-loss Conditions
Improves Circulation of the Abdomen, Feet, and Hands
Aids Conception
Reduces Hair Loss

**Parts Used:** The root, fruit, rhizome, and seeds

**Practical use:** Tincture, infusion, tonic wine

**Safety Precautions:** Do not take angelica internally during pregnancy, as it can cause uterine contractions.

## BASIL
*(Ocimum basilicum)*

Although most people usually make use of basil for culinary, not medicinal purposes, this plant is quite the healer. A powerful traditional remedy for inflammation, colds, and even snakebites, basil has many different health uses. For those who care deeply for their skin, studies have found basil to be loaded with anti-aging properties that prevent skin from drooping or sagging.

When my aforementioned friend was pregnant, she suffered from severe nausea. Even today, years later, she still thanks me for recommending basil juice to her. It made her mornings bearable, and after using basil for a time, she was able to enjoy food again.

**Native to:** India

**Description:** Basil is an herb you'll find used in kitchens all over the world, but it has also been shown to have a tremendous effect on our overall health. Extensively grown in Central and South America, and as a potted plant throughout the world, basil is an aromatic, annual herb of the mint family. Depending on the species (holy, sweet), the taste of the leaves varies, but they are all used for similar medicinal purposes. The key benefit of this plant is that it lowers blood glucose levels, so it is a common supplement for regulating diabetes. Sweet basil, in particular, has powerful therapeutic properties and is quite successful in easing nausea.

**Main Components:** Flavonoids, volatile oil, triterpene, saponins, polyphenols

**Medicinal Actions:**
Analgesic
Adaptogenic
Anti-inflammatory
Therapeutic
Antispasmodic
Anti-aging

**Main Uses:**
Lowers Blood Sugar
Reduces Fever
Relieves Nausea
Treats Stomach Cramps
Supports Digestion
Tonic to Improve Vitality
Relieves the Skin from Insect Bites

**Parts Used:** The aerial parts (that grow above ground)

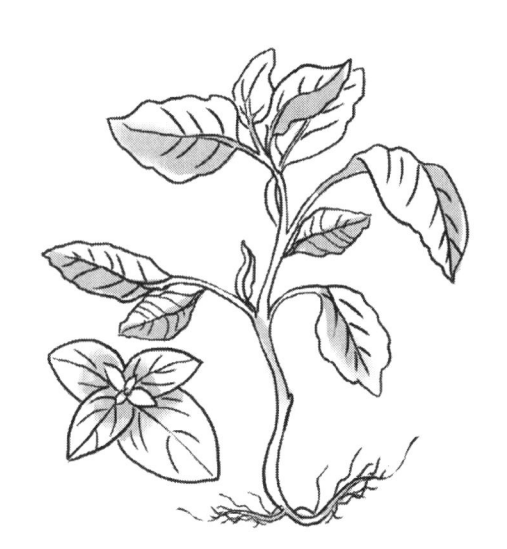

**Practical use:** You probably already use this in your culinary recipes but you can also make a basil tonic, juice, powder rub or a decoction.

**Safety Precautions:** Basil extracts and oils can slow down blood clotting. Avoid consumption if suffering from a bleeding disorder, as well as before and after surgeries.

# BLACK COHOSH
*(Cimicifuga racemosa)*

The popular Eclectic physician of the 19th century, John King, used to teach his students about black cohosh, his favorite remedy. Primarily known as "macrotys," black cohosh was the key remedy in Eclectic practices for treating chronic rheumatoid conditions.

Although I haven't had the chance to explore fully the benefits of this herb myself, my mother swears to its efficiency. She has been suffering from kidney issues her whole life, and she claims that black cohosh tincture is what keeps her out of the hospital.

**Native to:** Eastern USA, Canada

**Description:** Black cohosh is a powerful Native American supplement that has been used for women's conditions, such as menopause and painful menstrual cycles, for a long time. The root of the plant is the only part that is used and, although the taste is acrid and bitter, this natural remedy is still popular for treating kidney and rheumatic issues. You can find black cohosh growing widely and wildly in Europe, thanks to its seed propagation. You can also find this plant under the name of "black snake root" or "rattle top."

**Main Components:** Isoflavones, triterpenes, isoferulic acid

**Medicinal Actions:**
Sedative
Anti-inflammatory
Estrogenic
Antirheumatic
Expectorant

**Main Uses:**
Used for Treating Menopausal Symptoms
Relieves Painful Periods
Treats Rheumatoid Arthritis and Other Similar Issues
Treats Tinnitus (Ringing in the Ears)
Supports Kidney Health

**Parts Used:** The root

**Practical use:** Try making tinctures, decoctions, or tablets according to the chapter "Harnessing the Essence of Herbs."

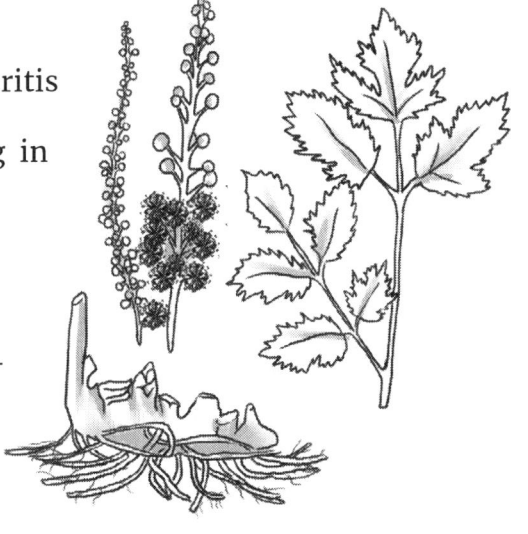

**Safety Precautions:** Avoid during pregnancy and if suffering from hormone-sensitive conditions. Black cohosh is known to work in a similar way to estrogen, and it can negatively impact female hormonal conditions such as endometriosis, uterine and ovarian cancer, fibroids, etc.

## CATNIP
*(Nepeta cataria)*

If you own a cat, then you probably are aware of this herb and the effect it has on your feline buddy – it makes cats roll, flip, growl, meow and, in the end – zone out. With a slightly different but also sedating intensity, this herb also affects humans. An old hangman's tale tells of how calming and relaxing the effect of catnip is. To endure his profession, the hangman used to drink a catnap (pun intended) tea before work, so he would not struggle as much with the ethical dilemma of his profession.

When my daughter was little, I used to give her catnip tea to restore balance to her colicky and upset tummy. This was especially beneficial if consumed around bedtime, as it used to promote a good night's sleep. For both of us!

**Native to:** Europe

**Description:** Born in Europe but naturalized in North America, catnip is an aromatic herb that commonly grows in higher-altitude and wayside areas. It has heart-shaped leaves and white flowers with purple dots. The flowering parts are used for medicinal purposes, mostly for settling an upset stomach or providing relief from colic. Thanks to its mild and non-bitter taste, catnip is good for treating infant, child and adult colic, anxiety, stress headache, and stomach trouble. It is also excellent in fighting colds and fevers because it encourages sweating. Sweetened with some honey, it can make a safe sedating remedy for children.

**Main Components:** Tannins, iridoids, volatile oil

**Medicinal Actions:**
Soothes Nerves
Encourages Sweating
Sedative
Relaxant
Anti-inflammatory
Spasmolytic
Antidiarrheal
Carminative

**Main Uses:**
Relief from Indigestion
Relief from Colic and Cramping
Reduces Fever, Cold, Flu
Treats Headaches
Lowers Anxiety
Reduces Rheumatism-related Pain when Applied as a Rub

**Parts Used:** The aerial parts (that grow above ground)

**Practical use:** Works perfectly as a tea, tincture, tonic, rub and compress.

**Safety Precautions:** Considered possibly unsafe for children, when taken in large doses. Should not be taken during pregnancy or breastfeeding. Avoid if planning on taking anesthetics or if suffering from pelvic inflammatory disease.

# CHAMOMILE
### *(Chamomilla recutita)*

Both Roman and German chamomiles are popular herbs used for their therapeutic properties. But there is a lot more than meets the eye with these well-known flowers. They do much more than simply soothe the nerves. I have found out that the herb penetrates deeply below the skin's surface, when applied topically, which makes chamomile an excellent anti-inflammatory agent.

If I don't savor a hot cuppa of chamomile tea before going to bed, I feel I cannot fall asleep. It relaxes and soothes me deeply, which is especially appreciated on those hectic days when all I want to do is unwind.

**Native to:** Europe

**Description:** German chamomile is one of the most widely used natural remedies. It is easy to cultivate as it is not demanding and thrives in temperate conditions. Chamomile has been the go-to natural supplement for herbalists in many eras, thanks to its soothing and relieving properties. The sweet, aromatic, white flowers with yellow centers offer an apple-like taste, perfect for tea. Roman chamomile is a closely related herb that offers similar medicinal benefits.

**Main Components:** Volatile oil, coumarins, flavonoids, bitter glycosides

**Medicinal Actions:**
Relaxant
Anti-inflammatory

Carminative
Antispasmodic
Antiallergenic

**Main Uses:**
Treats Indigestion
Relieves an Upset Stomach (bloating, acidity, gas)
Promotes Sleep

Eases Muscle Cramps
Eases Menstrual Cramping
Relieves Hay Fever and Asthma
Externally Useful for Itchy or Sore Skin

**Parts Used:** The flower heads (fresh or dried)

**Practical use:** A warm tea is very suitable. Even tinctures, essential oils and creams are great choices.

**Safety Precautions:** German chamomile is generally safe for everyone, but there are some precautions. Birth control pills, estrogen, and sedatives all interact with chamomile, so avoid using them together, or consult with your physician.

## CHICKWEED
*(Stellaria media)*

Chickweed is one of the most popular folk medicines. Well-known herbalists used to recommend it for treating skin conditions, pulmonary diseases, and as a remedy for mange (a parasitic skin disease). For the Ainu, the indigenous people of Japan, it was a go-to herb for bruises and bone aches. Although there isn't much scientific evidence to back this up, herbal enthusiasts swear by its incredible effects. Chickweed is bursting with iron, so it makes a great supplement for those suffering from anemia.

When my daughter was three years old, she was overcome by a severe case of eczema. She had struggled with itchy skin before that as well, but this was especially irritating. I didn't buy any conventional creams to relieve her itchiness. Instead, I used my homemade chickweed remedy and applied it daily. Not only did we manage to relieve her itchiness, but we also reversed the condition within a week.

**Native to:** Europe, Asia

**Description:** Small perennial with white flowers, oval leaves, and hairy stems. Although generally perceived as troublesome, chickweed is often found growing in wastelands and is quite a beneficial herb. Loaded with anti-inflammatory properties, this natural supplement is mainly used for treating irritated skin and, in some cases, extreme itchiness. Be mindful that, if consumed in larger quantities, chickweed can induce vomiting and cause diarrhea.

**Main Components:** Flavonoids, triterpenoid saponins, vitamin C, carboxylic acids

**Medicinal Actions:**
Anti-inflammatory
Emollient
Soothing Ointment
Anti-obesity Actions

**Main Uses:**
Treats Irritated Skin
Reduces Itchiness
Relieves Eczema, Nettle Rash, Venous Ulcers
Used for Baby's Diaper Rash
Relieves Stomach and Bowel Issues
Reduces Rheumatic Inflammation
Helps Maintain Weight

**Parts Used:** The aerial parts (the parts growing above ground)

**Practical use:** Makes a great cream, bath infusion and tea.

**Safety Precautions:** Generally safe to consume, but in medicinal amounts only. In high doses, chickweed causes vomiting and nausea. Avoid during pregnancy.

## DANDELION
*(Taraxacum officinale)*

Did you know that the milky white part of the dandelion stalk produces natural latex? During WW2, when the world was facing shortages in rubber supplies due to all the military needs, the world was forced to start looking for a natural alternative. And they found that alternative in dandelions. Or in their white sap, to be precise. But while your body may not have much use for dandelion latex, know that the same milky juice is quite effective for treating skin infections such as ringworm or eczema.

I absolutely love dandelion! In addition to making tablets and tinctures, I love incorporating the leaves into salads for lunch. I often struggle with high blood pressure, so this is another thing that helps me keep it in check.

**Native to:** Europe, Asia

**Description:** Dandelion is more than just a fun flower for kids to blow floaties. It is loaded with beneficial properties that support our health. Growing almost everywhere in the world and normally considered by the population to be a weed, dandelion is one of the easiest medicinal herbs to come by. Whether you choose to use the young leaves for a diuretic salad or harvest them later for tea, juices, or tinctures, this plant with yellow flowers, hollow stalks and basal leaves will cleanse your body from the inside out.

**Main Components:** Triterpenes, sesquiterpene lactones, polysaccharides, potassium – leaf and root. There are carotenoids and coumarins in the leaves, and phenolic acids, calcium, and taraxacoside hidden within the roots.

**Medicinal Actions:**
Bitter
Diuretic
Detoxifier
Anti-inflammatory

**Main Uses:**
Treats High Blood Pressure – leaf
Reduces Bodily Fluids – leaf
Stimulates the Liver – leaf
Treats Constipation – root
Reduces Local Inflammation – root
Treats Eczema – root
Good for Arthritic Issues – root
Stimulates Insulin Production – root

**Parts Used:** The root and leaves

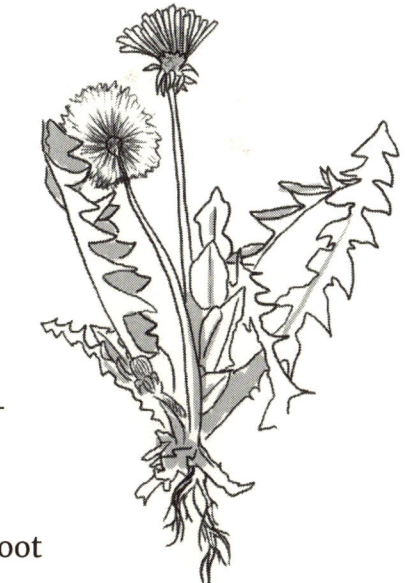

**Practical use:** You can go almost any route you wish with the easily found and very beneficial dandelion! My suggestions are tonics, juices, teas, tinctures, tablets, and consumed raw in salads (leaf only).

**Safety Precautions:** Generally safe, but in medicinal doses only. People with eczema are at higher risk of being allergic to dandelion, so do your due diligence before consuming. Also, dandelion is known to interact with antibiotics and can change the way that certain antibiotics react in the body.

# ELDER
*(Sambucus nigra; Sambucus canadensis)*

If you search the mists of 19th- and 20th-century folklore, you will definitely encounter elder. People believed that the Elder Mother, the elder guardian in Scandinavian and English folklore, inhabited the elder tree, so they always approached it with respect when gathering their medicines.

Today, elderflowers and elderberries still support our health in many mystical and magical ways. A couple of elderflower tea cuppas a day is my go-to remedy for slaying annoying seasonal allergies. Start consuming it a few months before the season hits, and you might lower your sensitivity and the severity of your allergies.

**Native to:** Europe

**Description:** You can find elder trees in most parts of Europe, thriving in the woods and in open areas. Its flowers and berries are loaded with medicinal properties that can relieve us from respiratory issues, purge cold and flu, and even support the removal of waste products by encouraging sweating and increasing urine production. If you dry the berries and make a decoction, you've got yourself a mild natural laxative. There are two black-berried varieties used medicinally: *S. nigra*, native to Europe and *S. canadensis*, native to North America. Both have the same uses.

**Main Components:** Flavonoids, tannins, anthocyanins, volatile oil, triterpenes, mucilage

**Medicinal Actions:**
Anti-inflammatory

Antiviral
Diuretic
Cleanses Mucus

**Main Uses:**
Treats Respiratory Infections
Lowers Cold and Flu Symptoms
Reduces Allergy Symptoms
Encourages Sweating
Controls Diabetes
Lowers Blood Pressure

**Parts Used:** The flowering tops and berries

**Practical use:** Make a tincture, tea, infusion or cream, depending on your needs and your mood.

**Safety Precautions:** Elderberries are considered not suitable for children younger than 12 years old. Elderflowers can cause vomiting and nausea if taken in high doses, and they can also interact with diabetes medications.

# FENNEL
*(Foeniculum vulgare)*

Fennel is one of the three main herbs used in the traditional, often banned, Absinthe recipe. It is also one of the nine herbs that were sacred to the Anglo-Saxons, the Germanic peoples who inhabited England in the 5th century. During medieval times, fennel was used to keep bad spirits away; this may or may not have been successful but, regardless, fennel still boasts powerful insect-repellent qualities.

Speaking of repellants, fennel is the perfect remedy for purging bad bacteria from the gut and one of the most effective natural digestive aids. My husband, who often struggles with digestive issues, benefits especially from fennel tea. He drinks a cup every couple of days as a preventive measure. I also used a fennel infusion as an eyewash when I was going through an annoyingly itchy allergy.

**Native to:** Mediterranean

**Description:** Cultivated in all temperate regions throughout the world, fennel is an aromatic plant with feather-like leaves, yellow flowers, and oval seeds. You've probably used these ingredients in cooking. When it comes to digestion, these little oval goodies, packed with volatile oil, work like magic. Apart from treating stomach-related issues, fennel seeds are also beneficial when used as an eyewash or for relief from conjunctivitis.

**Main Components:** Volatile oil, coumarins, sterols, flavonoids

**Medicinal Actions:**
Digestive Aid
Carminative
Antispasmodic

**Main Uses:**
Treats Bloating
Stimulates Appetite
Increases Breast Milk Production
Relieves Stomach-Related Issues in Infants, in Low Doses
Relieves Conjunctivitis
Relieves Menopausal Symptoms
Supports Weight Loss

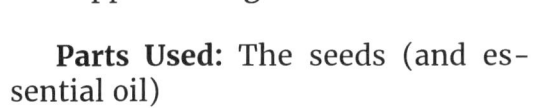

**Parts Used:** The seeds (and essential oil)

**Practical use:** Treat yourself with teas, capsules, tinctures, infusions and try fennel in culinary dishes.

**Safety Precautions:** Avoid with estrogen and birth control pills.

## GINGER
*(Zingiber officinale)*

Ginger has been one of the most popular herbs for medicinal and culinary purposes; there has been a consistent demand for the plant throughout the centuries. The first record dates back to

Confucius, who was known to eat this fragrant Indian staple with every meal. If you suffer from indigestion, you may want to consider doing the same, as studies find ginger to be quite effective in the stomach-emptying process (Bodagh et al., 2019).

A gingery infusion is my go-to morning drink. I have been drinking this for years to boost my immune system and support my weight maintenance goal.

**Native to:** Asia

**Description:** Ginger is more than just an aromatic staple in Asian cuisine. Rich in a volatile oil and packed with a pungent lemony taste, the rhizome of this plant is a must-have supplement for anyone looking for a natural approach to treating health issues. Thanks to its warming and stimulating properties, ginger has many medicinal uses. Supporting digestive health and relieving migraines and headaches are among the most common ones.

**Main Components:** Volatile oil, oleoresin

**Medicinal Actions:**
Anti-inflammatory
Digestive Stimulant
Circulatory Stimulant
Antiviral
Anti-emetic

**Main Uses:**
Supports Iron Absorption, Good for Anemia
Treats Indigestion and Supports Gastric Emptying
Reduces Muscle Pain
Relieves Morning Sickness and Motion Sickness
Relieves Symptoms of Spondylosis
Improves Circulation in Feet, Hands
Remedy for Chilblains
Remedy for Flu, Cough, and Respiratory Problems
Controls Fevers
Relieves Headaches

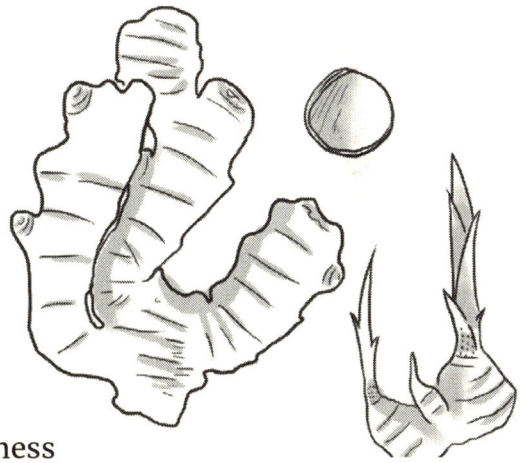

**Parts Used:** The rhizome

**Practical use:** One of my favorites, on a cold winter night, when made into a heartwarming tea. But also useful as infusions, tinctures, capsules, and essential oils.

**Safety Precautions:** Ginger is safe for both internal and external use. However, since it increases the risk of bleeding, this plant interacts with medications that reduce blood clotting and should not be taken along with such drugs.

## GINKGO
*(Ginkgo biloba)*

The ginkgo, the only living species in a genus of ancient, extinct trees, is in high demand as an herbal supplement. In early times, it was the magic bullet for improving memory and other age-related issues. Scientific evidence suggests that ginkgo may slow down the progression of Alzheimer's disease (Salleh, 2014), although that is not all this wonderful plant can accomplish. Ginkgo is most beneficial if used for glaucoma or blood circulation issues.

When my cousin's son was diagnosed with asthma, I suggested they give him a ginkgo remedy when the symptoms intensified. They say that he started feeling better after the first couple of sips. I haven't tried this myself, but many people claim that ginkgo has an incredible effect on asthmatic patients.

**Native to:** China

**Description:** It is believed that the ginkgo species is more than 190 million years old and that it is actually the oldest type of tree on earth. Although the therapeutic leaves have been an age-old medicine in native China, their beneficial properties have been made known to the world more recently. Research into this beautiful tree is just beginning. Ginkgo is one of the few herbs that crosses the blood-brain barrier (Liang et al., 2020) and this is the reason it is able to improve memory and circulation in the brain. It is also used as a relief from wheezing.

**Main Components:** Flavonoids, bilobalides, ginkgolides

**Medicinal Actions:**
Anti-inflammatory
Tonic for Circulation
Anti-allergenic
Antispasmodic
Anti-asthmatic

**Main Uses:**
Reduces Phlegm
Relieves Wheezing
Improves Blood Circulation, Especially to the Brain
Relieves Asthmatic Symptoms

**Parts Used:** The leaves and seeds

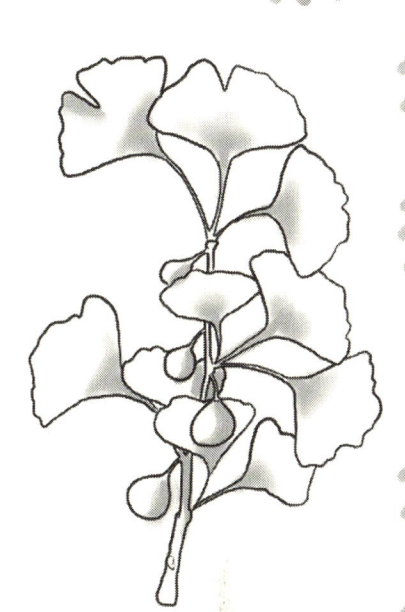

**Practical use:** Try tonics, tinctures, decoctions, fluid extracts and tablets to see what suits your body best.

**Safety Precautions:** Ginkgo leaves are safe to consume in appropriate doses, but the seeds are not recommended for internal consumption. Consuming more than ten seeds can cause a weak pulse, serious difficulty in breathing, shock, and seizures. Not safe during pregnancy and not recommended if taking Ibuprofen, as it can slow down blood clotting.

## GINSENG
*(Panax gInseng)*

If you visit the Geumsan region in South Korea, you may hear a 1500-year-old tale about a boy named Kang. When praying for his ill mother on Mount Jinak, a guardian spirit told Kang to look for a plant with three red fruits, take it home, and feed his mother the root. Soon after feeding his mother the root, the magical tea got his mother out of bed. The plant, as you may have guessed, was ginseng. Kang devoted his life to cultivating this magical plant and, in doing so, paved the region's path to becoming Korea's largest source of ginseng.

A dear friend of mine had liver cell damage (non-alcoholic fatty liver disease) and managed to reverse the condition within a couple of weeks by drinking ginseng tea every day. I wonder whether Kang's mother suffered from the same illness. Regardless, studies support that this herb has a great effect on the liver.

**Native to:** North and South Korea, Northeastern China, Eastern Russia

**Description:** As one of the most popular Chinese perennial plants, ginseng has been used as an herbal medicine for thousands of years. Difficult to cultivate and rarely found in the wild, this plant's root not easy to get your hands on. However, if you can manage to find it, ginseng can bring you tons of benefits. Excellent at improving stamina, ginseng is a popular supplement among athletes. It also serves as a male aphrodisiac. Although it is mainly used in Western societies for reducing stress, ginseng is also a powerful weapon for boosting the immune system and liver function.

**Main Components:** Panaxans, triterpenoid saponins, sesquiterpenes, acetylenic compounds

**Medicinal Actions:**
Tonic
Adaptogen
Stimulant
Hormonal Balancer

**Main Uses:**
Lowers Stress
Improves Stamina
Improves the Immune Function
Supports Liver Health
Reduces Nervousness and Anxiety

**Parts Used:** The root

**Practical use:** Ginseng works well in tonics, soups, and capsules.

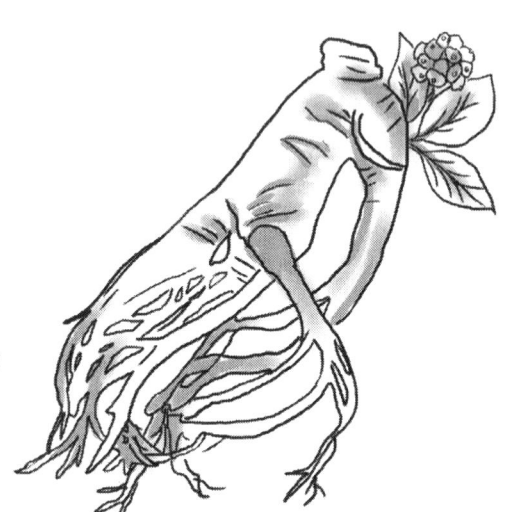

**Safety Precautions:** Avoid taking in combination with diabetes medications as it can affect blood sugar levels. Since ginseng can also raise blood pressure, avoid taking it in combination with caffeine. It also interacts with depression medications and Warfarin.

## GOLDENSEAL
*(Hydrastis canadensis)*

You may have heard the urban legend that consuming goldenseal before giving a urine sample can cover up the presence of recreational drugs. This probably stems from the 1900s novel Stringtown on the Pike, in which goldenseal causes false positives for strychnine poisoning. While I cannot comment on whether the writer, John Uri Lloyd, an herbal pharmacist himself, knew that this was only a myth, scientists had already dismissed the urban legend. Goldenseal can help you detox from cannabis, but it may not help you pass a drug test. Goldenseal will actually support metabolic flushing, which will lead to more THC in the urine.

When late fall rolls over, my annual sinus complications arise. When I was younger, I used to struggle with infusions and inhalations until I discovered that goldenseal extract was actually the most beneficial cure. I start consuming goldenseal in late summer and, as summer rolls along, I do not notice a single intense symptom.

**Native to:** North America

**Description:** This old Cherokeean remedy, goldenseal, was known as the cure-all herb for the Native Americans in the 19$^{th}$ century. The traditional use of this plant involved combining it with bear fat and applying it to repel insects, but it was also perfect for treating ulcers, wounds, and sores. Today, goldenseal is a rare and even endangered species that has many different practical uses. Goldenseal is perfect for stimulating the uterine muscles, thanks to the high alkaloid content, but is equally effective in lowering fat levels and maintaining a glucose balance in the blood.

**Main Components:** Isoquinoline alkaloids, resin, volatile oil

**Medicinal Actions:**
Tonic
Antibacterial
Uterine Stimulant

Anti-inflammatory

**Main Uses:**
Stops Internal Bleeding
Reduces Heavy Menstrual or Postpartum Bleeding
Stabilizes Blood Glucose
Remedy for the Mucous Membrane (Eyes, Nose, Throat, Ears, Stomach)

**Parts Used:** The rhizome

**Practical use:** This one is perfectly fine as a tincture, infusion, powder, decoction and capsules. Capsules can keep for a long time, without becoming spoiled.

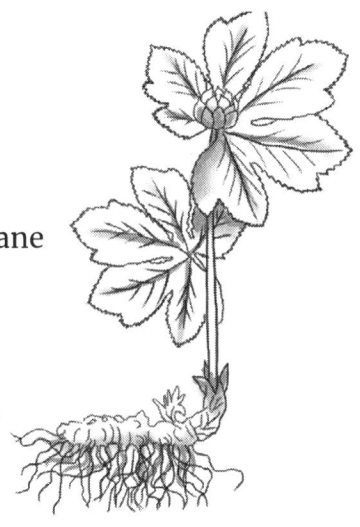

**Safety Precautions:** Not recommended for children or during pregnancy and breastfeeding.

## HAWTHORN
*(Crataegus spp.)*

Humankind has a long-standing bond with this plant. It extends from meeting fairy queens by hawthorn bushes, to the legend of Jesus' uncle planting the Holy Thorn of Glastonbury in Britain, and to the British Queen who decorates her Christmas table each year with a Holy Hawthorn sprig. It is known to soften the heart and be perfect for healing from grief. But that is not why it is known as "food for the heart." Studies suggest that hawthorn is the ideal natural supplement for reducing oxidative stress and is the best aid for supporting the cardiovascular system (Wu et al., 2020).

*I frequently consume hawthorn tonic for lowering blood pressure. I'm not a big fan of its bitter taste, but I can swear by its effect on normalizing the old ticker.*

**Native to:** Great Britain

**Description:** This tree sports red berries and grows along roadsides. Oftentimes, the plant is mistakenly considered poisonous.

Although it doesn't taste great in a berry parfait, it will surely energize the cells of your heart. Primarily, it is used for treating angina or heart irregularities, thanks to its power to dilate and relax the arteries. It is equally effective for improving memory and the blood flow to the brain, especially when taken in combination with ginkgo.

**Main Components:** Coumarins, polyphenols, bioflavonoids, triterpenoids, amines, proanthocyanins

**Medicinal Actions:**
Antioxidant
Circulatory Tonic
Cardiotonic

**Main Uses:**
Lowers Blood Pressure
Reduces Angina Symptoms
Increases Blood Flow to the Muscles
Increases Blood Flow to the Brain
Treats Coronary Artery Diseases
Great for Normalizing Heartbeat

**Parts Used:** The flowering tops and berries

**Practical use:** Aim for a decoction, tonic, tincture, infusion or make tablets.

**Safety Precautions:** Not recommended for those who take heart medications. It can also interact with drugs for high blood pressure, so consult with a physician before using it. Avoid during pregnancy and breastfeeding.

## HOPS
*(Humulus lupulus)*

First used for brewing beer in the 16th century in England, this herb was considered by the parliament of that time as "the wicked herb." Since becoming an integral ingredient in one of the most consumed beverages on Earth, scientists have started exploring the effects this herb has on our health over time (Kyrou et al., 2017). And the results don't lie! Hops can be quite beneficial. Consume hops regularly, and you will not have problems falling asleep, or with anxiety.

I drink hops infusions when I need to unwind mentally. I don't usually suffer from insomnia but, when I do, I can be up and turning all night, unable to fall asleep. When this severe condition pays me a visit, I brew myself some hops tea, add a dash of valerian to it, and sleep like a baby.

**Native to:** Europe, Asia

**Description:** You may not have seen climbing hop plants often, but you have surely tasted this herb many times before. Hops give beer its bitter and characteristic taste. The hop plant is a member of the *cannabis* family, and hops have similar sedative and sleep-inducing properties. They can also help relax your muscles and even bring an estrogenic effect.

**Main Components:** Volatile oil, bitters, flavonoids, estrogenic substances, polyphenolic tannins

**Medicinal Actions:**
Sedative
Antispasmodic
Contains Aromatic Bitter Compounds
Soporific

**Main Uses:**
Treats Insomnia
Lowers Excitability
Relaxes Muscles
Stimulates the Digestive System
Reduces Tension and Stress

**Parts Used:** The strobiles (the conelike female flowers)

**Practical use:** Use in an infusion, tincture, sachets, or craft into tablets and capsules to harvest the benefits you desire.

**Safety Precautions:** Avoid if suffering from depression, before and after surgery, with alcohol, and with sedatives.

# LEMON BALM
*(Melissa officinalis)*

With the reputation of being able to lift the spirit and heal the heart, lemon balm was the ultimate "youth elixir." Being one of the key ingredients in cordials, a soft, diluted drink consumed during medieval times, this herb was very popular among royalty. The Prince of Gamogan, a county in Wales, used to drink lemon balm tea every day and actually lived for 108 years!

I don't know whether it will help us all live to be well past 100, but I can surely attest to lemon balm's amazing medicinal properties. I use it as a tonic for relieving aching flu symptoms, and it always manages to boost my spirits.

**Native to:** Europe, Northern Africa, Western Asia

**Description:** If you have lemon balm in your herbal garden, then you know how this lovely aromatic plant is adored by the bees. Once you experience its calming properties yourself, you will enjoy it just as much. From providing a sense of relaxation when you're feeling down, to relieving cold sores, to helping you restore your overactive thyroid function, this fragrant herb will definitely find its purpose in your home apothecary.

**Main Components:** Flavonoids, volatile oil, tannins, polyphenols, triterpenes

**Medicinal Actions:**
Relaxant
Carminative
Nerve Tonic
Antispasmodic
Antiviral, Especially for Herpes
Hormonal Herb

**Main Uses:**
Treats Overactive Thyroid
Relieves Cold Sores
Relieves Anxiety
Reduces Panic and Nervousness
Relieves Flu Symptoms

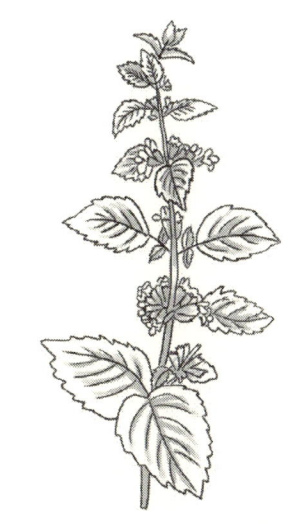

Treats Insect Stings

**Parts Used:** The aerial parts (the parts that grow above ground)

**Practical use:** A very popular tincture, infusion, essential oil, juice, lotion, or ointment, when needed.

**Safety Precautions:** Generally safe for everyone, but avoid if suffering from thyroid disease, as lemon balm is known to change the thyroid functioning.

## LICORICE
*(Glycyrrhiza glabra)*

Did you know that licorice's main compound, glycyrrhizic acid, is 50 times sweeter than sugar? That is why if you look up 'candy' in a thesaurus, you'll find it synonymous with licorice. Apart from its sugary taste, the root of this plant is one powerful herbal medicine. In fact, a two-year study found that licorice extract is more effective for treating GERD (Gastroesophageal Reflux Disease) than conventional antacids (Setright, 2017).

My husband suffers from heartburn, so wherever he eats foods that upset his stomach, like orange juice or tomatoes, I prepare him a tincture which he consumes an hour after the meal. It feels very satisfying when all of his symptoms mysteriously disappear.

**Native to:** Europe, Southwest Asia

**Description:** Licorice root is one of the most effective herbal remedies. It is jam-packed with powerful anti-inflammatory properties, but it is also a powerful anti-arthritic herb. It supports the treatment of many conditions, from heartburn and arthritis to canker sores. It also serves as a gentle laxative to help battle constipation. In addition, licorice stimulates the adrenal glands. With all these uses, you don't need to feel guilty about picking up some licorice from the candy store again.

**Main Components:** Isoflavones, phytosterols, triterpene saponins, polysaccharides

**Medicinal Actions:**
Anti-inflammatory

Demulcent

Mild Laxative
Adrenal Agent
Anti-arthritic

**Main Uses:**
Treats Inflammatory Digestive Conditions
Treats Addison's Disease and Other Adrenal Issues
Relieves Arthritic Symptoms
Treats Menopausal Symptoms
Helps with Inflamed Joints
Soothes Inflamed Eyes

**Parts Used:** The root

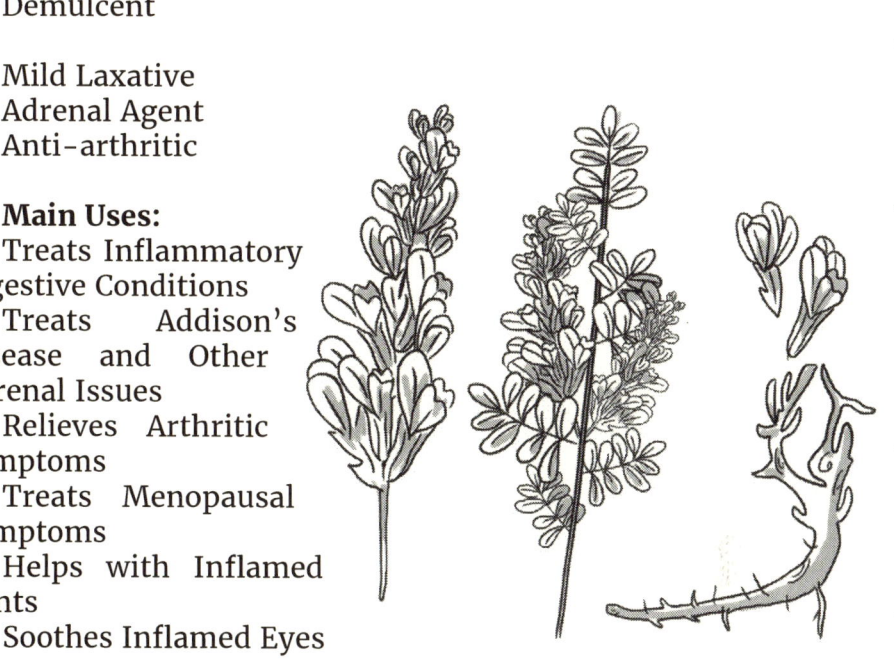

**Practical use:** Bring out the goodies with a tincture, powder, extract or a decoction and you won't regret it.

**Safety Precautions:** Avoid during pregnancy as significant amounts of licorice increase the risk of early delivery. Also, avoid if suffering from high blood pressure, if you have hypertonia (a muscle condition), kidney problems, or you are taking Warfarin.

## MILK THISTLE
*(Silybum marianum)*

The medicinal use of milk thistle can be traced back to the first century; and in Roman times, herbalists referred to this plant as the "carrier of bile" or the plant that could cleanse the internal fluids. Now a popular liver remedy in Western herbal medicine, many studies have backed up the efficacy of milk thistle (Mulrow et al., 2000).

My dear college friend made a life-threatening mistake when camping in Germany as a student. She and her boyfriend consumed death cap mushrooms thinking they were edible. Fortunately, just as their friend was about to put the grilled shroom in his mouth, he noticed that something was odd. He put two and two together and realized that the mushrooms they had just been grilling were incredibly deadly. They immediately went to the hospital and, two hours later, they received a medication with silymarin as a base. Silymarin is the extract from the seeds of milk thistle, and it protects the liver. It prevents highly toxic compounds from causing permanent damage to the liver and kidneys.

**Native to:** The Mediterranean

**Description:** Milk thistle can be found throughout Europe and now also commonly occurs in California. It is a spiny plant, with pink flowers, that thrives in sunny and open areas. It is mainly used for treating liver conditions, especially when the cells need to be renewed. It is a powerful remedy for hepatitis but is also perfect when the liver is under stress, such as during chemotherapy. As the name suggests, milk thistle also induces breast milk production.

**Main Components:** Flavonolignans, polyacetylenes, bitters

**Medicinal Actions:**
Liver Protective
Anti-allergenic
Chemoprotective
Anticancerous

**Main Uses:**
Treats Liver Conditions
Treats Jaundice and Hepatitis
Supports Liver Function During Chemotherapy
Increases Breast Milk Production
Relieves Symptoms of Allergic Rhinitis

**Parts Used:** The flower heads and seeds

**Practical use:** A traditional herb which is frequently used in tinctures, decoctions, tablets, and capsules. And it's easy to imagine why, what with all its uses.

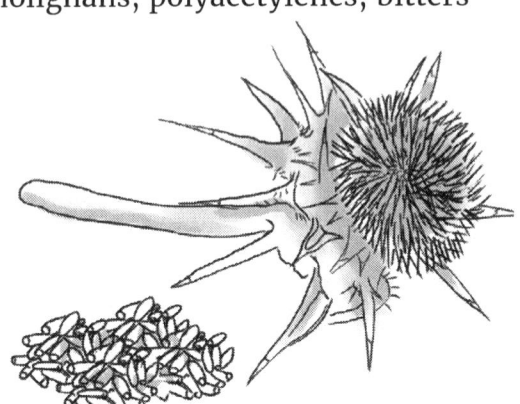

**Safety Precautions:** Avoid during pregnancy. Use only in appropriate doses, as a large amount of milk thistle can cause bloating, gas, nausea, and upset stomach. Avoid with hormone-sensitive conditions such as endometriosis or fibroid cancer, as milk thistle extract mimics estrogen.

## NETTLE
*(Urtica dioica)*

Derived from the word "needle" and translated from Latin as "burn," this herb can inflict painful stings, as many people already know. But, aside from its sting, nettle can also give great healing to its users. It has various health benefits, but nettle's most recognized clinical action is its protection against benign prostatic hyperplasia (Ghorbanibirgani, 2013).

When I was pregnant with my daughter, I had severe iron deficiency. My OB told me that I would never be able to retrieve the normal iron levels with just herbs, and not stronger medications; I managed to prove him wrong. Among other herbal supplements, my main iron booster was my yummy nettle-leaf soup.

**Native to:** Temperate regions all over the world

**Description:** If you haven't felt a nettle's sting, then it is clear you are not spending enough time in nature. Leave the comfort of your home! Stinging nettle leaves have a long history of being quite the healer. This plant's anti-inflammatory and anti-allergenic compounds offer powerful protection from fever, arthritis, and anemia. Nettle is a cleansing and detoxifying herb that everyone should have in the herbal home apothecary. It is sought after, not only for its leaves, but also for its roots, which have just as many beneficial medical compounds trapped inside them.

**Main Components:** Amines, flavonoids, minerals, glucoquinone; phenols and sterols (root only)

**Medicinal Actions:**
Anti-inflammatory
Diuretic
Astringent
Anti-allergenic
Tonic

Prevents Hemorrhaging

**Main Uses:**
Increases Urine Production
Stops Bleeding from Wounds
Treats Nosebleeds
Treats Asthma and Hay Fever
Protects Liver Function
Relieves Arthritic Symptoms
Treats Enlarged Prostate Symptoms (the root)

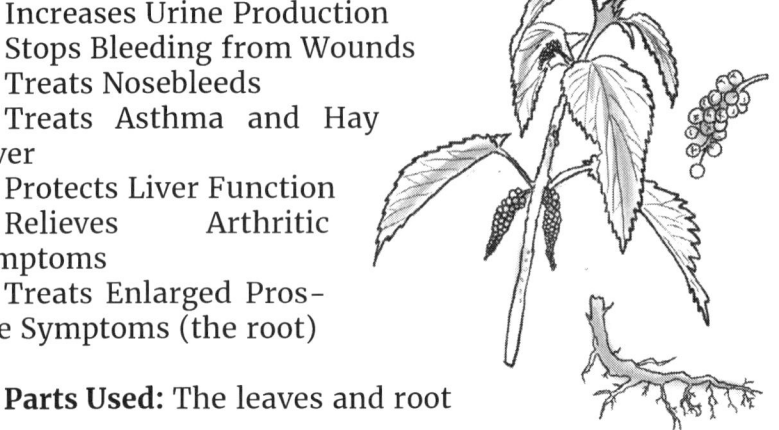

**Parts Used:** The leaves and root

**Practical use:** Usually used in tinctures, decoctions, soups, infusions, ointments, and capsules, depending on your needs. Refer to the chapter "Harnessing the Essence of Herbs" if you are having trouble creating one of these from nettles.

**Safety Precautions:** Avoid during pregnancy, as nettle can cause uterine contractions. Also, keep in mind that medication for diabetes interacts with nettle, as the plant also has glucose-lowering properties.

## PEPPERMINT
*(Mentha x piperita)*

Just how old a cure is peppermint? History tells us that dried leaves were discovered in Egyptian pyramids. Clearly, Egyptian royalty thought peppermint wasn't only great for life, but for the afterlife as well. It is now 3000 years later, and we still depend on this powerful and fragrant herb for many conditions. Large clinical studies confirm that peppermint is an invaluable cure for treating irritable bowel syndrome (Chumpitazi et al., 2018).

After my C-section with my daughter, I struggled with bloating and gas, a common side effect from the abdominal operation. Peppermint tea and essential oil are packed with so many therapeutic properties that I was able to eat solids much sooner than I had anticipated.

**Native to:** Europe, North America, Asia

**Description:** Peppermint is more than the aromatic in your mojito. It is a powerful herbal medicine that carries with it a strong therapeutic effect. Rich in volatile oils and acting as an antibacterial, peppermint has a cooling effect on inflamed skin. It is also a powerful antiseptic. Its forte is treating digestive issues and giving pain relief, especially in the abdominal area. When peppermint essential oil is rubbed on the temples, it can also alleviate headache symptoms.

**Main Components:** Volatile oil, phenolic acids, flavonoids, triterpenes

**Medicinal Actions:**
Antiseptic
Antibacterial
Antispasmodic
Analgesic
Carminative
Antimicrobial
Stimulates Sweating

**Main Uses:**
Relieves Bloating, Gas, and Colic
Treats Digestive and Bowel Issues
Relaxes the Gut Muscles
Reduces Skin Sensitivity
Treats Eczema
Relieves Nausea
Soothes the Colon
Relieves Diarrhea
Relieves Pain (Especially Abdominal Pain and Headaches)

**Parts Used:** The aerial parts (that grow above the ground)

**Practical use:** A world-renowned herb which I use frequently when eating foods that produce gas, like legumes. Fine as infusions, teas, essential oils, ointments, and capsules. Keep in mind that this herb has many other uses similar to the ones mentioned above.

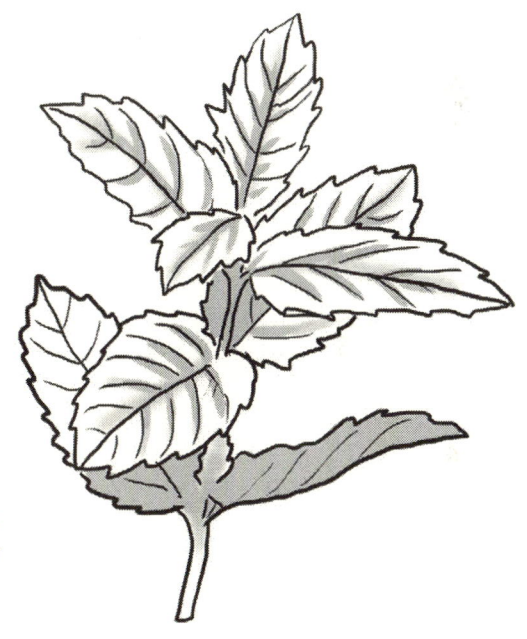

**Safety Precautions:** Peppermint is generally safe for everyone. However, those suffering from diarrhea should avoid peppermint, as the herb can cause unpleasant anal burning. Peppermint also relaxes esophageal sphincters, which can make heartburn and GERD worse.

# ROSEMARY
*(Salvia rosmarinus)*

With a ton of folklore uses and even more medicinal purposes, rosemary deserves a special place in your herbal kit. Its main benefit is memory improvement, which is why many students (especially in the Mediterranean) used to burn rosemary sprigs when studying for exams.

My relationship with rosemary started in the kitchen but I soon found a much better use for this natural and aromatic herb. My rosemary tincture has guided me through many stressful situations. When I feel the pressure piling up, I release steam by mixing 40 drops of rosemary extract with a glass of water. Whether I am on a time crunch, trying to get work done for a project, or simply trying to finish my chores, rosemary is great for circulating blood to my head. It also lifts my spirits.

**Native to:** The Mediterranean

**Description:** Though it is one of the most used herbs in the world, rosemary does more than just enhance your culinary delicacies; it improves your health as well. Rosemary makes a warming tonic that soothes the nerves, promotes healthy blood flow, stimulates the adrenal glands, and uplifts the mood. It helps battle stress and mild depression, can ease rheumatic muscles, and increases concentration. It is perfect for circulation, especially for people with low blood pressure.

**Main Components:** Volatile oil, tannins, rosmarinic acid, flavonoids, diterpenes

**Medicinal Actions:**
Anti-inflammatory
Stimulant
Nervine

Tonic
Antioxidant
Astringent

**Main Uses:**
Improves Concentration and Memory
Relaxes the Nerves
Relieves Stress and Tension
Raises Blood Pressure
Supports Circulation
Relieves Mild Symptoms of Depression
Relieves Headaches
Supports Hair Growth
Relieves Aching Muscles

**Parts Used:** The leaves

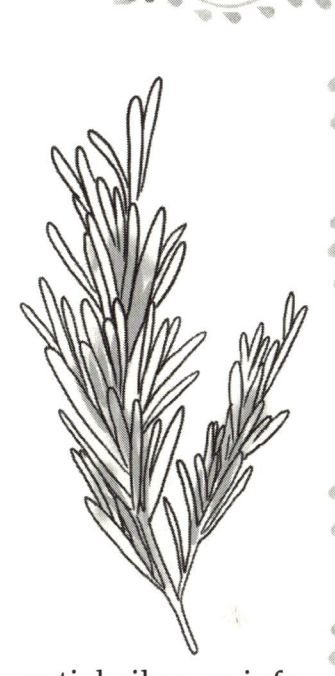

**Practical use:** Prepare it as a tincture, essential oil or an infusion, and it won't disappoint.

**Safety Precautions:** Safe if eaten, but should be avoided during pregnancy. Consume in appropriate doses as a high amount of rosemary causes kidney damage and stomach irritation. Avoid if you are allergic to aspirin.

# SAGE
*(Salvia officinalis)*

Sage was a crucial part of the ancient Roman pharmacopeia. Romans used it frequently to support the digestion process after consuming fatty cuts of meat, popular at that time. Today, sage is often used as a preservative for meat, but that is not why this herb has found its way onto this list. Sage has a vast array of medicinal properties; the greatest of which is its antiseptic character. Hildegard of Bingen, a German Benedictine abbess, visionary, prophet, and herbalist who lived just over 900 years ago, famously said, "Why should a man die whilst sage grows in his garden."

A few months back, we were visiting some friends who had just moved to their farmhouse. The property was full of animals, had beautiful, lush gardens, and insects buzzing from flower to flower. While there, my daughter received a strange sting on her hand, that wasn't from a bee or a mosquito; unfortunately, my herbal kit was nowhere to be found. I looked around my friend's garden and saw sage among the herbs. I picked a few leaves and started rubbing them onto the sting site. Five minutes later the irritation was gone!

**Native to:** The Mediterranean

**Description:** As the meaning of its botanical name suggests (*salvere*; to be saved), sage does not only do wonders for our pork or our holiday meals, it also transforms our health. It is a powerful antiseptic, and effective in regulating hormonal activity. It is particularly helpful for hot flashes. Sage is a must-have herb for women in their 50s. There is also strong support for sage's beneficial effect on our nerves, but one of the most popular uses today is as a remedy for sore throats.

**Main Components:** Essential oil, tannins, diterpenes, phenolic compounds, triterpenes

**Medicinal Actions:**
Astringent
Estrogenic
Antiseptic

Nerve Tonic

**Main Uses:**
Sore Throat Gargles
Digestive Tonic
Relieves Menopausal Symptoms
Supports Regular and Normal Menstrual Cycle
Lowers Blood Fat Levels
Decreases Depression Symptoms
Enhances Memory
Relieves Bites and Stings

**Parts Used:** The leaves

**Practical use:** Prepare as a tincture, infusion, or tea.

**Safety Precautions:** Not recommended during pregnancy, as it contains thujone, a chemical that induces the menstrual cycle.

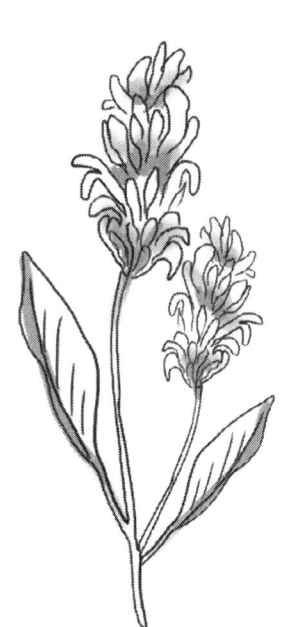

Sage also lowers blood sugar and can interact with medication for diabetes. It can also interact with seizure drugs.

## ST. JOHN'S WORT
*(Hypericum perforatum)*

St. John's Wort has recently been revived as an herbal remedy, in all its medieval glory! Although we can no longer say that it protects us from evil influences, a belief of many medieval people, this yellow summer flower brings dozens of medicinal uses to your home apothecary.

My dear friend, who was suffering from postpartum depression, took a St. John's Wort tincture a couple of times a day and was able to overcome her mental hardships quickly. During the Middle Ages, this flower was believed to cure insanity and, though people no longer suffer from "general insanity," this herb is still extremely useful for treating mental exhaustion.

**Native to:** Temperate Regions Throughout the World

**Description:** These summer yellow flowers not only look good in your vase, but they can also do wonders for your mental well-being. Known as one of the most powerful herbal antidepressants, St. John's Wort is a nerve tonic that restores and keeps our mood in check. Still, that's not the only way we benefit from these lovely flowers. St. John's Wort is also excellent for repairing tissue, and its oil is one of the most effective alternative medicines for post-surgery recovery.

**Main Components:** Flavonoids, phloroglucinols, polycyclic diones

**Medicinal Actions:**
Antidepressant
Anti-inflammatory
Anxiolytic
Antiviral
Tissue Repair

**Main Uses:**
Treats Depression Symptoms
Calms the Nerves

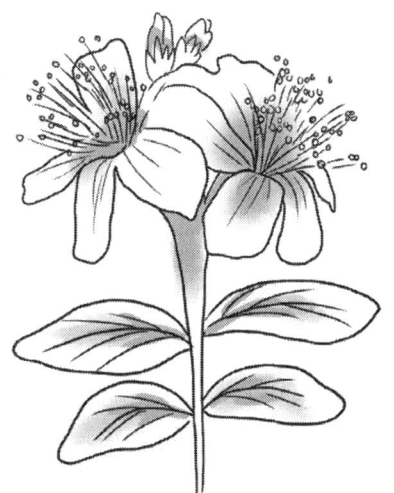

Lowers Anxiety
Promotes Recovery After Surgeries
Heals Wounds and Burns
Improves Lowered Mood During Menopause

**Parts Used:** The flowering tops

**Practical use:** This is one of the herbs best used fresh, to make tinctures, infusions, infused oils, and creams.

**Safety Precautions:** Not recommended during pregnancy as some studies suggest it causes birth defects. Also not recommended during breastfeeding as it can cause colic and drowsiness in infants.

## TURMERIC
### *(Curcuma longa)*

This Indian cuisine staple offers more than a bit of spice or a dash of yellow color to your meals. It is one of the most powerful and oldest medicinal foods in existence. Every herbal healer should keep a hefty supply of turmeric around. Records of turmeric's use for medicinal purposes date from more than 4,000 years ago.

Although the therapeutic actions of this golden spice started gaining attention only a few decades ago, every alternative medicine aficionado will confirm that having turmeric in your home apothecary is a must. And I am here to attest to its incredible anti-inflammatory properties. I have Hashimoto's disease, which is an autoimmune illness of the thyroid, and taking my turmeric tincture with water is what keeps the paths of inflammation clear.

**Native to:** India, Southeast Asia

**Description:** This most valuable remedy in Indian culture has spread throughout the world in recent decades, and for good reason! Turmeric is a powerful medicinal agent that can support and improve our health in many different ways. It has shown benefits, from fighting inflammation to lowering cholesterol (Hewlings & Kalman, 2017). It is a key ingredient in beating chronic health issues. The yummy golden powder and its main constituent, curcumin, have unparalleled medicinal use.

**Main Components:** Curcumin, resin, volatile oil, bitters

**Medicinal Actions:**
Anti-inflammatory
Antimicrobial
Lowers Cholesterol
Antiplatelet

**Main Uses:**
Fights Inflammation
Relieves Allergies
Treats Autoimmune Diseases
Supplement for Dementia, Diabetes, and Cancer
Lowers Cholesterol Levels
Keeps the Blood Thin
Protects the Stomach and Liver by Increasing Bile Production
Beneficial for Gastritis
Assists with Eczema, when Applied to the Skin

**Parts Used:** The rhizome (broken, boiled, and then dried)

**Practical use:** Turmeric is used as a tincture, powder, and decoction. I often personally use the powdered form in my soups. I use it when cooking as it gives that beautiful golden color to white meat and vegetables. It also smells divine!

**Safety Precautions:** Generally safe, but not recommended for people suffering from gallbladder conditions. It also interacts with anticoagulant medications.

# VERVAIN
### (Verbena officinalis)

Vervain is one of the most popular "magical" herbs. But despite its contribution to witchcraft and ritual ceremonies, it has also left an incredible mark on the scientific world and on the history of herbal medicine.

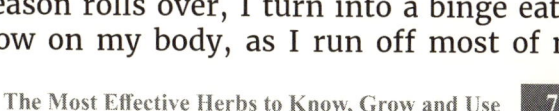

When the holiday season rolls over, I turn into a binge eater. Although it doesn't show on my body, as I run off most of my calories, trust me when I tell you that I can eat a lot. Last Christmas, there were so many leftovers (I not only binge eat, but binge cook as well) that I thought swallowing them up was the best way to prevent my hard work from going to waste. A couple of hours later, my tummy ached like a toddler's after eating too many candies. A vervain infusion did the trick and helped relieve all the pressure in my stomach. Vervain helps the digestive system absorb food quickly and restores gut balance!

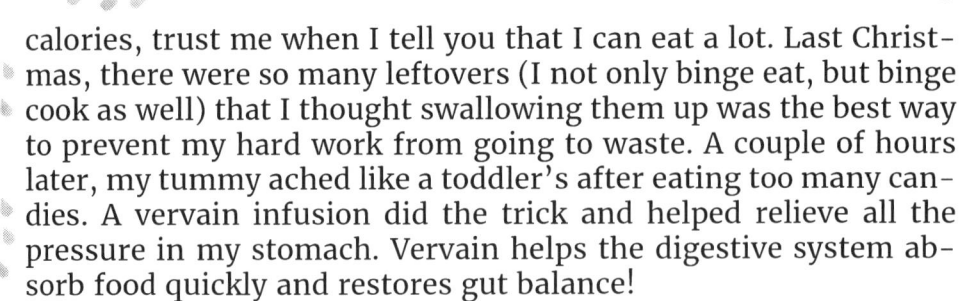

**Native to:** Southern Europe

**Description:** Acting as a cure for nearly every ailment throughout the centuries, vervain is a versatile herb with many medicinal properties. Its uses stretch from stimulating the womb, to supporting digestion and dealing with headaches. It also does wonders for our nervous system. It is safe to say that, whatever health issue you're dealing with, there is certainly some benefit that vervain can bring your way. If none of these reasons is enough to convince you to add vervain to your herb garden, consider that it can also be used as toothpaste! Powdered vervain rubbed on the teeth and gums can keep them clean and protected.

**Main Components:** Flavonoids, alkaloids, bitter iridoids, volatile oil, triterpenes

**Medicinal Actions:**
Mild Antidepressant
Nervine
Tonic

**Main Uses:**
Deals with Digestive Issues
Relieves Nervous Tension
Good for Reducing Depression Symptoms
Tonic for Chronic Illnesses
Relieves Headaches and Migraines
Relieves Premenstrual Syndrome

**Parts Used:** The aerial parts (that grow above ground)

**Practical use:** This herb is commonly prepared as a tincture, infusion, and powder.

**Safety Precautions:** Generally recognized as safe, but not recommended during pregnancy.

# YARROW
*(Achillea millefolium)*

Did you know that Achilles, a hero of the Trojan War in Greek mythology, shares his name with this white flower? In fact, it is thought that these white flowers helped this Greek legend heal his wounds on the battlefield. Whether Achilles was named after the herb, or the herb has gotten the name thanks to the way it helped heal him heal, is up for a debate. But what's certain is this: yarrow is a heavenly herb for healing.

When my husband cut his arm on one of our frequent outdoor adventures, I applied yarrow poultice onto the cut and wrapped it up tightly. When we got home, we were both surprised to see how very little blood there was. While that was my first experience of yarrow in action, I can definitely attest that Achilles was right – applying yarrow on wounds will keep them clean and stop blood flow.

**Native to:** Europe, North America, Western Asia

**Description:** With similar healing properties as chamomile, yarrow is another essential herb you should never be without. With tons of powerful constituents that bring incredible health benefits, it is no surprise this plant has a long-standing reputation among herbalists. Yarrow minimizes external and internal bleeding; it dilates the blood vessels, has antitumor properties, and it is also powerful in fighting against the common cold and flu by encouraging sweating and reducing the fever.

**Main Components:** Flavonoids, volatile oil, alkaloids, sesquiterpene lactones, tannins, triterpenes, phytosterols

**Medicinal Actions:**
Bitter Tonic
Astringent
Anti-inflammatory
Antispasmodic
Mild Diuretic

Stops Bleeding

**Main Uses:**
Treats Wounds
Lowers Blood Pressure
Reduces Fever
Regulates Menstrual Flow
Decreases Cold and Flu Symptoms
Tones Varicose Veins
Helps with Digestive Infections

**Parts Used:** The aerial parts (that grow above ground)

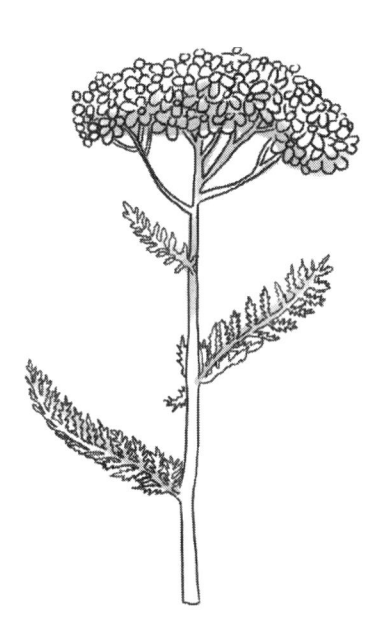

**Practical use:** Great for tinctures, essential oils, and poultices. This herb may help you greatly with digestive issues, wound healing, depression, and anxiety, and fighting inflammation; it truly is nature's gift. Then again, which herb is not?

**Safety Precautions:** Avoid during pregnancy and when breastfeeding. Yarrow also slows blood clotting and shouldn't be taken with anticoagulant medications.

All the previously mentioned herbs are loaded with helpful constituents that provide powerful medicinal actions. The trick to squeezing the most out of them lies in using them correctly. After adding these rich and powerful ingredients to your herbal magic kit, it is time to take the next step. It is time to learn how to start your own medicinal garden and make sure that you are equipped with the right tools for extracting the active ingredients. If you are ready to lay the foundations of your home apothecary, jump to the next chapter!

# Your Own Medicine Garden and Home Apothecary

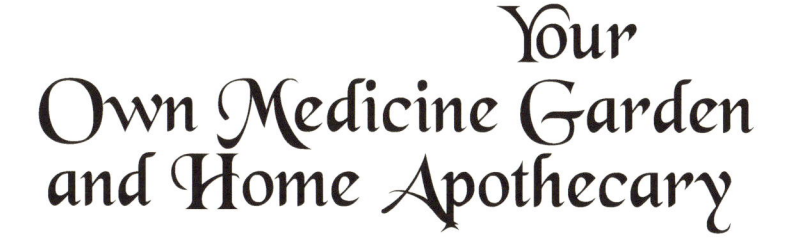

Now that you know what medicinal herbs you should take advantage of to support your overall health, the time has come to think about setting up your own home apothecary. In the ideal scenario, your home apothecary is also accompanied by a lush herb garden – a place that will allow you to gather the needed herbs for your remedies in the most convenient way possible. Let's face it though, most of us live under conditions that are far from ideal. The lucky ones who have settled in far-flung rural corners, surrounded by acres of land, can exploit and experiment with various plants, as they see fit. But should that mean that those living in small apartments are doomed never to try their hand at growing herbs? Definitely not!

Not all herbs demand large spaces or constant sunlight. Some actually thrive in a windowsill garden. So, whether you grow them next to a window, in a corner in your kitchen, on your balcony, or in a small backyard, anyone can hop onto the herb-growing bandwagon.

If you don't already have a medicinal herb garden, there are a few factors to consider before getting started:

**The Place** – Growing indoors, outdoors, or under a cover (such as inside a greenhouse) will all require slightly different approaches.

If you plan on cultivating the herbs in your backyard, choose hardy plants with roots that can penetrate deeply, and with lush foliage that will provide a plentiful harvest. If the plants aren't hardy, you should think about moving them someplace sheltered.

If planting indoors, choose a hanging basket, container, window box, or a small flowerpot for the herbs to do their magic. Extra precaution is needed when growing indoors, as herbs can dry out or outgrow their pots. If they are kept in conditions that are less than ideal, then the possibility of these events becomes all-the-more likely. Transplant to larger containers, when needed, to prevent the plants from becoming pot bound. Aloe vera, basil, calendula, chamomile, lavender, lemon balm, rosemary, sage, St. John's wort, thyme, and yarrow all thrive indoors.

If you have a greenhouse, then you have a few more options. You can tweak the growing conditions and adjust the temperature and humidity as you see fit, so it will be possible to grow a range of exotic and more "needy" herbs.

**The Sun Exposure** – Whether indoors or outdoors, there is one thing that all herbs require: proper sun exposure. Medicinal herbs thrive in sunny areas, so make sure to provide a proper place to nourish your sweet little plants. Inside, place the containers near the windows or someplace where they can get plenty of natural light. Outside, find sunny corners and avoid spots where larger plants, trees, or buildings cast shadows during the day.

**The Soil** – Most herbs need well-drained soil. If growing indoors, make sure to buy potting soil and never fill the containers with outdoor soil. Firstly, that soil is a lot heavier and, more importantly, it can contain bacteria and diseases that can eventually kill your indoor herbs.

If growing outdoors, make sure to analyze the soil first and establish that it is a healthy growing medium. Take handfuls of soil, gathered from different spots in the garden, and check them with a soil test kit, which is available from most gardening stores. Check the soil pH and see what kind of compost will be best to enrich the soil. Most medicinal plants require a pH of 6.3–6.8.

Once you take care of the essentials, you should then decide whether to cultivate from seed or buy your medicinal plants from an herb nursery. If choosing the latter, pay attention that you buy standard medicinal plants, as many herbs are improved and sold mainly for ornamental purposes.

**Proper Maintenance** – Immediately after planting, you should give your plants and seeds enough water to kickstart healthy growth. After that, it is probably wise to water your herbs only once or twice a week, rather than water them every single day. Remember, the point is not to overwater, as the medicinal actions are the greatest when the conditions are drier.

When it comes to feeding the herbs, keep in mind that giving mulch or other fertilizers to your medicinal plants may lower their potency and therapeutic properties. However, that doesn't mean that you shouldn't treat the soil before planting. The soil must be nutritious enough to provide a healthy environment for the herbs.

If your plants are diseased or infected, separate them from the healthy ones, and treat with organic cures only. A good solution may be to soak garlic in water and then spray it over the plants in order to repel pests.

# Harvesting and Processing

Whether you have your own garden or are an outdoor aficionado like me, and love the thrill of looking for herbs in the wild, proper harvesting and processing are crucial for the quality and intensity of the medicinal actions of the plants.

## Harvesting from the Wild

The wild offers an abundance of free medicinal herbs. Harvesting herbs in the wild makes you feel truly connected with nature and with the inner herbal-healing instincts that you possess! But what I love most about this harvesting method is that wild-grown herbs are more concentrated than those found in your home garden. That means that wild medicinal plants will have a more powerful effect on your health than the herbs growing in containers in your home. However, as appealing as this sounds, there are quite a few concerns you need to pay attention to:

*Identification* – I cannot stress this enough! Proper identification is essential. Improper identification can possibly be life-threatening. It's easy to mistake a harmful wild plant for some medicinal herb. For instance, poisonous foxglove leaves are often mistaken for comfrey. So, before you head out to the great, wild woods with your rucksack in tow, make sure you know your herbs well, as misidentification can easily lead to serious problems.

*The Site* – You may be tempted to harvest nettles that grow by the road, but I strongly suggest you rethink that urge. Plants growing near roadsides, factories, or even fields where the crop might be sprayed with pesticides, should most certainly be avoided. Instead, try to go deep in nature, far from sources of pollution or other areas where plants may be in contact with artificial materials.

*Other Ecological Factors* – Never harvest more plants than you plan to use. In addition, do not uproot wild herbs; instead, make a clean cut with a sharp knife or scissors. Keep in mind that bark shouldn't be collected from the wild, as stripping this layer from the tree can put the whole plant at risk.

When harvesting in the wild, place the cut herbs inside a nylon sack and make sure not to pack them too tightly together.

## Harvesting from Your Garden

If you're cultivating your own garden, then you have medicinal herbs always at your fingertips. All you have to do is simply gather what you need. But as simple as it sounds, there is actually more to harvesting herbs than just cutting them with a pair of scissors. It must be done with gentle, tender care, as being too rough with these precious herbs may put the entire plant's chance of survival at risk.

Here are the four steps to harvesting properly from one's garden:

**#1 Gather the Right Equipment** – The most important part of harvesting herbs is to do so with a clean cut. It is also vital that you avoid crushing the herbs you have cut. I recommend a pair of sharp scissors and an open tray or basket.

**#2 Harvest at the Right Time** – It goes without saying that you should harvest your plants at peak maturity to ensure the highest concentration of beneficial compounds. As a general rule, herb plants gain strength towards the time of flowering; many are strong enough to use all season, but they are strongest just before flowering. Leaves are best harvested just before budding. Flowers are best harvested when most are still in the bud stage, but a few have opened. If you wait, the flowers will be pollinated, and their properties then diminish rapidly, sometimes in only a few days. At this stage, the plant puts all its energy into developing seeds. Fruits and berries can be harvested when they become ripe, and the root can be collected in autumn, or when the plant starts drawing the nutrients from the aerial parts into the ground parts.

**#3 Harvest the Right Parts** – Keep in mind that different parts of the plant have different medicinal actions. Do your due diligence before harvesting, to make sure that the collected herbs will address your condition properly.

**#4 Harvest the Right Amount** – Never gather more than you need, period. If you're not about to process, or not planning to use the herbs immediately after harvesting, do not collect as many. If using for salads or cooking, the herbs are best consumed right after harvesting. If making remedies, it is recommended that you process them as soon as possible.

## Preserving the Harvested Herbs

Did you know that aromatic herbs lose the majority of their powerful volatile oils only a few hours after being harvested? That's why processing the harvested herbs at a low temperature, and as quickly as possible, is crucial in order to prevent the medicinal compounds from deteriorating rapidly.

There are many ways in which you can process the herbs to preserve their active constituents, but the easiest and simplest of all is by letting them dry naturally in the air, or by popping them into a cool oven to dry for a bit of time.

### Stems and Leaves

When harvesting stems, make sure to separate the flowers and large leaves from the bunch, as they should each be processed in a slightly different way.

The stems and smaller leaves should be gathered in a bunch of eight to ten. Then it is important to secure with them with some strand – not too tightly, as there should be room for air circulation between the stems and leaves. Hang them upside down in a dark and warm place that is not too hot and has good ventilation. If the air is very humid, use artificial heat like your oven or a dehydrator for the drying process. Check in on the herbs daily, and when the stems and leaves become brittle, but not so dry that they crumble, they're ready. Grab a tray or a piece of newspaper and rub the stems with both your hands to separate the small leaves.

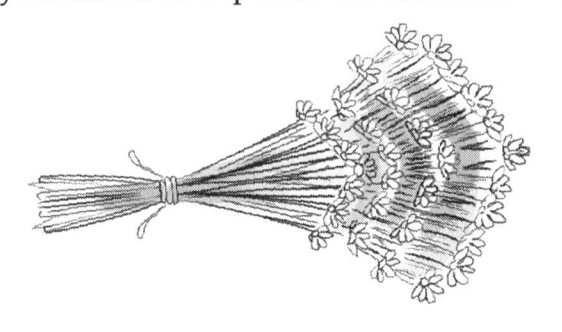

### Flowers

For large flowers, separate them immediately after harvesting, and inspect well to remove any insects. Line a tray with a piece of absorbent paper and arrange the flowers in a single layer on the tray. Then place the tray in a warm, dark, well-ventilated spot.

Smaller flowers can be harvested while still attached to the stalk and then hung in bunches, just like stems. With flowers, I suggest putting them in a paper bag first and then securing them with a strand.

If you plan to use only the petals, and not the whole flower head, be sure to remove the petals before storing; then discard the heads.

### Berries and Fruit

Fruits and berries should be harvested when they reach peak ripeness, not only because they are the most effective at that stage, but also because they may not dry properly if overripe.

Arrange them on a tray lined with absorbent paper, and pop inside a warmed oven. The oven should not be on – just warm. Do not close the oven door. Instead, crack it open, and let the fruits sit for about four hours. Then, move the tray to a warm and dimly lit place. Check the berries and fruits daily, turning them over occasionally, until they have dried out fully.

## Roots, Rhizomes, and Bulbs

After harvesting the plants' underground parts, you should wash them thoroughly to get rid of the dirt. Dry them with some paper towels. Chop the roots or bulbs finely; they will dry faster if small, and most become rock hard after drying. If there are any damaged parts, discard them.

Just as with the berries, place the chopped roots onto a tray lined with absorbent paper, place in a warmed oven with the door open, and allow to sit for a couple of hours. Then move the tray to a dark and warm area, and keep it there until the roots are completely dried.

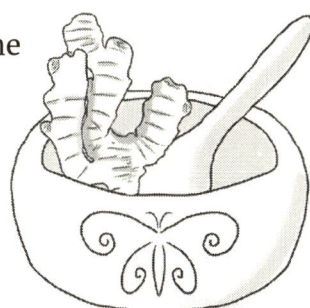

## Seeds

Gather the seed heads into small bunches, tie them together, and hang them upside down in a warm, dark, well-ventilated place. If the seeds are tiny, you can place the heads in a paper bag before tying them together. When dried, gently shake them inside the bag, to help free the seeds from the heads.

## Bark

As I've mentioned before, gathering bark from the wild is not a good idea as a plant that loses its bark will die. However, if you already have your own medicinal shrubs, you can harvest the beneficial bark from outlying branches, with extra care and love. Later, you can prune back those areas with minimal damage done to the plant.

Chop the bark up finely, arrange on a tray, and place in a dark and warm area to dry in the air.

## Gel and Sap

Harvest gel and sap with care and only while wearing gloves, as the milky juices can often be corrosive. You can collect these liquids by squeezing the stems over a bowl. If gathering aloe vera gel, you can do it by cutting the leaves lengthwise and then peeling the edges off.

Gel and sap do not need to be processed, as they already are in their medicinal forms.

## Storing the Herbs

If not stored properly, your herbs will not last. Be sure they are completely crisp dry before storing, as the slightest bit of moisture will allow mold to grow. Once they are dried, you can place them in sterilized, opaque glass containers with air-tight lids. Alternatively, you can choose a more inexpensive option and store them in new and unused brown paper bags. Be cautious when using the paper bag method of storage because your herbs will require an especially dark and dry place for storage. Keep in mind that the lifespan of your brown-bagged herbs is much shorter. Air-tight storage is much more effective; herbs in air-tight jars can last a full year after harvesting, while those in brown bags only last about six months.

For gel and sap, if not using right away, you can simply pour the liquid into an ice cube tray and freeze for prolonged lifespan and convenient use.

*Important: Never store your herbs in plastic or metal containers, regardless of their quality. Metal and plastic can ooze chemicals that may contaminate the herbs.*

With your apothecary now full of dried herbs, let's learn how to use them and extract the trapped goodies inside, so you can address your health issues the natural way.

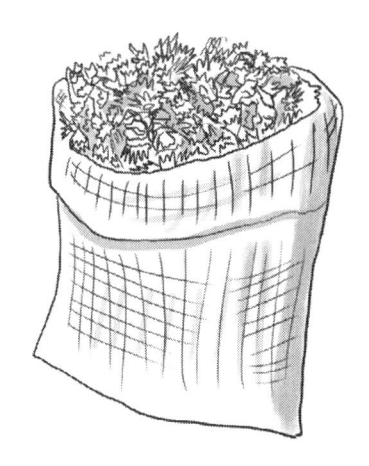

# Harnessing the Essence of Herbs

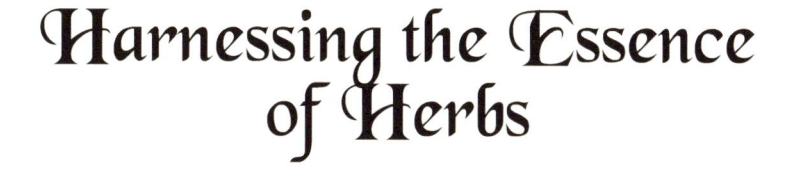

Even the most well-stocked home apothecary will not be beneficial if you fail to extract the medicinal properties out of the herbs correctly. Each of the plants mentioned in this book comes with valuable constituents, which are trapped in different parts of the plant. To become a real herbalist, it is your job to understand which parts provide the most important medicinal actions, and more importantly, how to extract the active components and turn them into a readily available medicine.

Nothing is better than munching on fresh herbs! However, this is inconvenient with modern life, doesn't work well with barks and doesn't preserve the herbs for the cold season. The following methods of extraction, chosen with each specific herb in mind, allow you to access everything potent in the plant all year round. This is something you cannot possibly achieve while simply munching on the leaves.

There are many different extraction methods: these include basic infusions, soaking in alcohol, extracting powders, and making topical applications. All of these methods will be covered in this herbal book. Herbal extracts come in the form of liquids, creams, powders, and oils, all of which contain substances that can address different health issues.

It may sound like a daunting task at this point but

you don't necessarily need extensive herbal knowledge or herbal family roots to harness the essence of the medicinal plants you've chosen to grow. All you need is the right guidance and clear instructions to follow, which are covered in this next chapter. So, hop on this herbal train and get ready for the magical act of whipping up herbal potions, creams, tinctures, and all sorts of mixtures that will do wonders for your health.

## Infusions

As the name suggests, infusion is a process in which the dried herbs are steeped in an absorbing liquid, water being the easiest one to use. The process is like making tea. Although tea is an infusion, not all infusions are tea. Often, it's alcohol that is used as the liquid to make a tincture, or oil that is destined for a salve. This is the simplest and most straightforward way to use the aerial parts of the plant for medicine. The only difference between brewing a tea for pleasure and one for medicinal purposes, is strength. A medicinal infusion is stronger, usually because of a longer steeping time, but sometimes also because of the amount of herb used. Tea is a more neutral and mellow drink, which is why it is widely enjoyed; infusions aren't normally so tasty.

To make a hot water infusion, normally just called an infusion, you will need:

- A Kettle
- A Tea Strainer
- A Cup with a Lid
- Your Herbs of Choice
- Hot Water

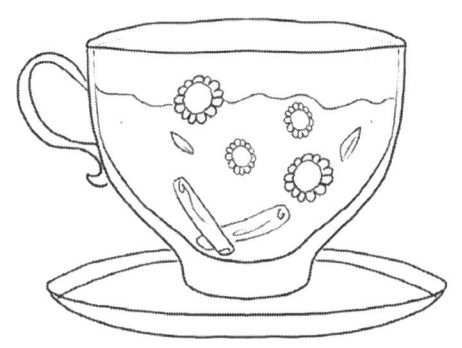

### How to infuse:

1. Boil some water in a kettle.
2. Place about a teaspoon of the preferred dried herb in a strainer.

3. Place the strainer inside the cup and pour the boiling water over the top of the herbs.

4. Cover the cup with a lid and let it steep for seven to ten minutes before removing the lid.

5. Remove the strainer with the herbs, catching the last precious drips of medicine.

6. Sweeten with some honey, if desired, and enjoy warm or cold.

Alternatively, you can perform an infusion in a pot. You will need:

- A Kettle
- A Pot with a Lid
- A Cup
- Hot Water
- Herbs of Your Choice
- A Mesh Strainer

## How to infuse in a pot:

1. Boil some water in the kettle and pour two cups of the boiling water inside the pot.

2. Add about 20 g (0.7 oz) of dried herbs and place the lid atop the pot.

3. Let sit for ten minutes.

4. Place the mesh strainer over the cup and strain the infusion into the cup.

5. Enjoy!

The key to making an infusion is to <u>cover the cup while steeping.</u> Most medicinal actions in the herbs are due to the presence of volatile oil, which can quickly be dispersed into the air if you're steeping without a lid.

Tip: To make herbal tea, the process is pretty much the same. Cut down the steeping time to five minutes, so that the tea isn't quite so potent. That's it!

Dosage: A standard dosage is to take about 3 cups of infusion per day. Of course, this varies from herb to herb, as some have a stronger taste and effect, while others can be quite refreshing (e.g., yarrow vs. chamomile). If the herb is quite intense and you decide to take a large dose, the infusion can end up having a negative effect.

Storage: Infused beverages can be stored in a covered pot, bowl, or jug in the fridge, for up to 24 hours.

## Cold Infusions

For some conditions, you may need to extract the herbs using a cold infusion. Some active constituents can be destroyed when introduced to heat; the process of infusing herbs in cold water is called cold infusion.

For a cold infusion, you will need:

- A Bowl
- A Fine-Mesh Strainer
- A Jug
- Water
- Herbs

Performing a cold infusion:

1. Combine the herbs and water in a clean bowl. For 25–30 g (about 1 oz) of herbs, I recommend 2 cups of water.

2. Let the mixture steep overnight.

3. Place the fine-mesh strainer over the jug and pour the contents of the bowl through the strainer and into the jug.

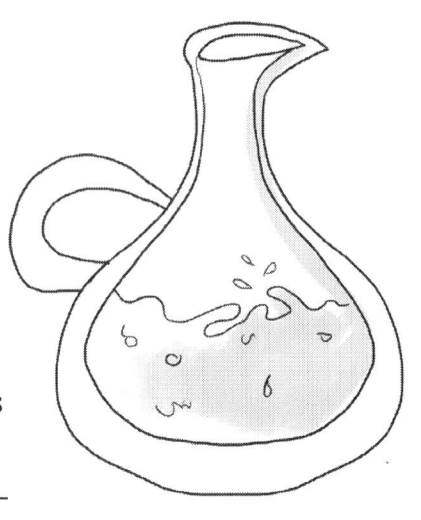

4. Consume a cold infusion as you would consume a hot water infusion or a decoction.

*Storage:* Cover and place in the fridge; consume within the next 48 hours.

## Decoctions

Not all parts of the plants can be easily infused. If you need to extract bark, roots, or berries, you will need a slightly stronger approach. Decoctions are a slightly more complex trick up an herbalist's sleeve but do not worry, you can make them too. Decoction is a process of extraction in which the herbs are simmered in boiling water.

In Chinese medicine, decoctions are the preferred method of extraction. Chinese herbalists make especially concentrated decoctions by adding many different herbs to the potion or simmering for a long time, until the liquid is reduced to less than a cup.

Decoctions are mainly used for drinking, but they are also effective if applied externally, such as for washes.

To make a decoction, you will need:

- A Saucepan
- A Jug
- A Mesh Strainer
- Herbs
- Water
- A Stove

How to make a decoction:

1. Place the herbs inside the saucepan. For a daily dosage, add about 20 g (0.7 oz) of dried herbs or 40 g (1.4 oz) of fresh ones. If using a mixture of herbs, go with 40 g (1.7 oz) in total.

2. Cover the herbs with cold water (3 cups for a daily dosage) and place them over medium heat.

3. Bring the liquid to a boil, then lower the heat and let simmer for 20–30 minutes. The strained liquid should be reduced from 3 cups to 2 cups in volume.

4. Remove the saucepan from heat.

5. Place the mesh strainer over a jug and pour the liquid through the strainer.

6. Consume as needed.

If the mood strikes you, you can also add more delicate parts to the decoction. If you think you will benefit more if you add some flowers, leaves, or stems to the mix, place them inside the pot, just after you turn off the heat. That way, they will start to infuse as the mixture begins to cool.

*Dosage:* Just as with the infusion, the right dosage depends on the herbal intensity but, for most plants, a daily decoction of 2 cups will do the trick. You can take a decoction warm or cold.

*Storage:* Cooled, leftover decoction can be stored in a covered pot or jug and refrigerated for up to 48 hours.

## Tinctures

Tinctures really pack a punch. Made by soaking herbs in alcohol, this extraction is probably the strongest method of all. Tinctures can be different strengths depending on the herb-to-alcohol ratio, and the strength of the alcohol used, among other factors. Alcohol is measured in terms of concentration (proof) and volume (liquid ounces, liters or milliliters), while herb content is measured in weight (grams or ounces).

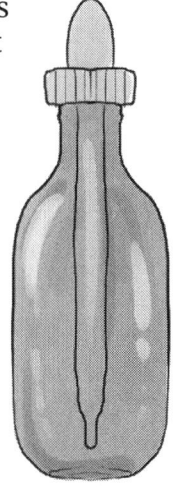

Tinctures are classified according to the ratio of herb to menstruum (solvent), with the menstruum being composed partly of alcohol, and partly of water. The aim, when making a tincture, is to end up with a final product that is at least 20% alcohol, so that the tincture is shelf stable. Most tinctures work well with vodka because that menstruum ratio is 40:60 (40 units of herb to 60 units of menstruum) or 50:50, and the active medicinal components are mostly water soluble. The alcohol concentration is high enough that the finished product is 20% (40-proof) or higher, ensuring that the tincture will be shelf stable.

If the herb being used is fresh, the juice and active components will be extracted out of the plant cells and will dilute the alcohol-water solvent. Thus, when making a tincture out of juicy leaves, for example, one must start with stronger alcohol, to allow for the extra dilution that will take place. Examples of these herbs are lemon balm and St. John's wort. When using a gum or resin, like myrrh, the alcohol needs to be near 95% (200-proof).

## Tips on alcohol amount and strength

80 to 90 proof vodka (40-45% ethanol content). Fill 40% to 50% alcohol by volume.
- The usual percentage range for tinctures.
- Suitable for fresh herbs with low moisture and dried herbs.
- Suitable for extracting water-soluble active components.

Half 80 proof (40% ethanol) vodka & half 190 proof (95% ethanol) grain alcohol. Fill 67.5% to 70% alcohol by volume.
- Suitable for extracting those volatile aromatic components.
- Suitable for fresh and juicy herbs. Berries, aromatic roots, and lemon balm for example.
- The stronger alcohol concentration will extract the plant juices.

190 proof grain alcohol (95% ethanol content). Fill 85% to 95% alcohol by volume.
- Suitable for extracting the aromatic components and essential oils that don't dissolve easily.
- Suitable for diffusing gums and resins but not necessary for other plant parts.
- This alcohol strength will dehydrate your herbs if botanicals other than gums and resins are being tinctured.

*Important: Never prepare tinctures with industrial alcohol, rubbing alcohol, or methyl alcohol!*

If you still find this a bit daunting, after doing your research on the specific herbs you wish to use and asking your herbalist friends, the Facebook group "Herbalism For Beginners At Home – Medicinal Herbs and Herbalist Remedies" is a great place to ask for guidance.

Although most popular in Western herbal medicine, tinctures also have a long, traditional use. These preparations are very convenient to use, can be prepared with pretty much any herb, and can be applied to treat a wide variety of health concerns.

To make a tincture yourself, you will need:

A Large Clean Jar with a Lid
A Muslin Bag (Nylon Mesh or Cheesecloth also Work Well)
A Large Pot (or Wine Press)
Small Dark Glass Bottles
A Funnel
Vodka
Preferred Herbs

How to create a tincture:
1. Place the herbs in a clean and sterilized jar, and pour the vodka over them. If using fresh herbs, you can go with a 1:2 ratio, adding double the weight of alcohol to your fresh herbs. If using dried herbs, though, the suggested ratio is 1:5. You should pour five times the weight of vodka into the jar as you have herbs.

2. With more potent herbs, the ratio could be 1:10 or even 1:20. Do prior research on the specific herbs and ask your herbalist friends, in order to determine a suitable herb-to-vodka ratio. Put the lid on, and secure tightly. Shake the jar well for a couple of minutes, then place it in a warm and dark place. (You can speed up the making of tincture with warmth – around 38ºC or 100ºF. Leave it there for about 10–14 weeks, making sure to shake the jar for a minute or two every couple of days.

3. When the time for straining comes, place the clean muslin bag over the large pot or wine press. If using a wine press, simply press it strongly to extract the tincture. If straining over a regular pot, just pour the jar contents carefully

through the cloth, then bring the edges of the cloth together, trapping the herbs inside, and squeeze to extract well. Alternatively, you can do this with a regular mesh strainer.

4. Using a funnel, carefully transfer the strained liquid into the sterilized dark glass bottles. Seal tightly!

5. Although vodka is the alcohol of choice for most herbalists, you can also use rum, especially if you include bitter herbs. The taste of the rum can mellow out the non-pleasing herbal taste.

*Dosage:* The standard dose is to take about a teaspoon of tincture diluted in about 1 ½ tbsp of water or juice, two or three times a day, depending on the herbs used.

*Storage:* Store the sealed dark glass bottles in a dark and cool place. Properly stored tinctures will remain safe to use for up to two years.

## Syrups

We grownups may be fine with drinking infusions and decoctions, but children are usually not big fans of these herbal remedies, especially if we're using unpalatable and bitter plants. And what better way to force them to take their medicine than with a sugary bribe? That's when syrups come to the rescue!

Syrups are made with equal amounts of infusion and honey or unrefined sugar. In addition to being sweet in taste, syrups also come with an added benefit; they bring an extra soothing action to the mix, which is why they are so effective for treating sore throats and coughs. Besides this, they are also jam-packed with sugar which is a natural preservative. This helps the infusion or decoction survive for months on the shelf.

The important thing to know about making syrups with infusions and decoctions is that the herbs must be infused for the maximum time for the maximum potency. If using an infusion, steep for a full 15 minutes, and if using a decoction, simmer for half an hour.

To make a syrup, you will need:

- A Saucepan
- A Wooden Spatula
- Dark Glass Bottles
- A Funnel
- Infusion or Decoction
- Honey or Refined Sugar
- A Stove

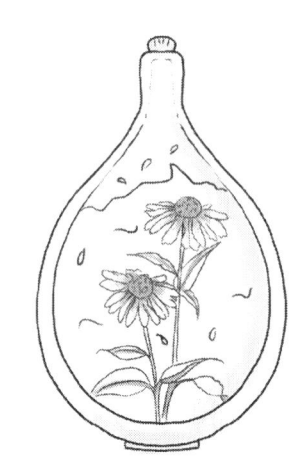

How to create a syrup:

1. Add about two cups of the prepared infusion or decoction into a saucepan.
2. Add the honey at this point – 500 g (17.6 oz) for 2 cups of infusion, or half the amount if only using 1 cup of infused liquid.
3. Stir over low heat, until the honey or sugar is fully mixed.
4. Turn off the heat and allow the saucepan to cool down.
5. Use a funnel and pour the syrup into dark, sterilized glass bottles.
6. Secure tightly and use the syrup as needed.

You can also make a syrup with a tincture. For this preparation, you will need:

- 500 g (17.6 oz) Honey or Unrefined Sugar
- 1 cup Water
- Tincture
- A Saucepan
- A Wooden Spatula

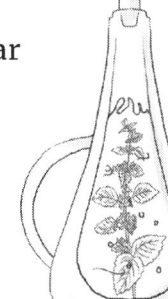

- A Jug
- A Funnel
- Dark Glass Bottles
- A Stove

To make a syrup with a tincture:

1. Combine the honey (or sugar) with the water in the saucepan.
2. Place over medium heat, and heat gently, stirring until the sugar or honey is dissolved.
3. Remove the saucepan from heat and allow the syrup to cool completely.
4. Place one part of your preferred tincture into a jug and add three parts of the syrup to it. If using ¼ cup of a tincture, add ¾ cup of the syrup.
5. Stir to combine and pour into your sterilized dark glass bottles with the help of a funnel.
6. Close and use the syrup as needed.

<u>Dosage</u>: Take about 1–2 teaspoons of the syrup, three times a day.

<u>Storage</u>: Store the dark glass bottles in a dark and cool place, and consume the syrup within the next six months.

## Infused Oils

You may be familiar with this method for adding a bit of flavor to your dishes, but infusing herbs in oil can be quite beneficial for your health as well. By infusing the medicinal plants this way, you encourage their fat-soluble constituents to be released. In the process, you unlock compounds that you otherwise cannot extract.

There are two oil infusion methods: hot infusion, by simmering herbs in oil over gentle heat; and cold infusion, by letting the herbs naturally and gradually release their goodies at room temperature. Since the beneficial compounds in herbs can break down at temperatures of above 100°C (212°F), so cold infusion is the preferred method.

When making infused oils, no drops of water should get into the oil. This can support microbial growth and ruin the infusion. For this reason, it is preferable to use dried herbs in your infusions. However, if you wish to use fresh herbs (which give a stronger flavor), you should first rinse the herbs to clean them, then pat with paper towel and leave overnight to dry and wilt completely in the air, before adding them to the oil. Hot infusions keep for longer, but cold infusions can still be stored in the refrigerator for several months. If you notice any unusual smell to your infusion, it has possibly become contaminated with bacteria or mold and should be discarded.

## Hot Infusion

Hot-infused oil can be used in many ways, from drizzling over meals for flavor, to applying by rubbing oil onto the skin for therapeutic massage and healing purposes. It can even be used as a secret ingredient in your ointments. You can use olive, sunflower, or any decent-quality vegetable oil for this purpose.

You will need:

- A Saucepan
- A Heat-Resistant Glass Bowl with a Lid
- A Wide-Mouthed Jug or Simple Pot
- A Muslin Bag or Cheesecloth
- A Dark Glass Bottle
- A Funnel
- Herbs
- Vegetable Oil
- A Stove

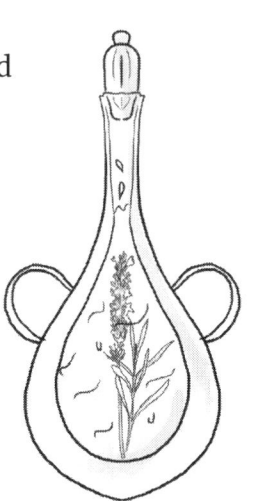

And here is how to do it:

1. Place about 1 cup (250 g or 8.8 oz) of dried herbs in a clean glass bowl.

2. Pour between 1¼ and 1½ C of oil over the herbs, and give the mixture a stir.

3. Fill the saucepan half way with water and place it over medium heat. Bring to a boil.

4. Place the glass bowl in the mouth of the saucepan, so that the base of the bowl is resting in the warm water. Cover the glass bowl with a lid, and allow to heat gently for at least a couple of hours. (Alternatively, you can use a double boiler for this.)

5. Keep the temperature of the oil between 38 and 60°C (100–140°F).

6. Remove the bowl from the heat and allow to cool until it is safe to handle.

7. Place the muslin bag over the wide-mouthed jug, tucking the middle of the cloth inside, while the sides remain over the jug, so there is no mess while pouring.

8. Pour the oil gently through the muslin bag. Bring the edges of the cloth together, trapping the herbs inside, and gently squeeze to extract the strained liquid into the jug.

9. With the help of a funnel, pour the strained oil into the previously sterilized bottle. Seal tightly and use as needed.

## Cold Infusion

Cold infusion is a much slower process, but it is the preferred method because it preserves the active compounds and gives a stronger flavor. Fresh herbs are usually used in a cold infusion, especially smaller flowers and other delicate parts of the plant. However, be careful to dry the herbs thoroughly before using them, as water will encourage the growth of bacteria and mold in the oil. It is best to leave the herbs in the air for 24 hours so that excess water can evaporate off. This extraction is encouraged by sunlight, and it is best done with olive oil, as it is the least likely to turn rancid.

However, it is worth mentioning that many herbs like lemon balm and St John's wort lose much of their benefits when dried. I use fresh, although wilted, herbs all the time.

A well-made oil has little or no water in it to grow mold. The problem is people are putting fresh herbs in oil and then sealing the jar. You should use dried herbs if you're going to do that. The right procedure with fresh herbs is to cover the top of jar with a coffee filter or cheese cloth then heat it or leave under the sun for up to 48 hours. It doesn't matter whether you choose to use the sun or artificial heat. I like my crockpot on the lowest to evaporate the water and infuse the oil. When you have taken this extra step with fresh herbs, strain, cap tightly and store in dark place.

Here is what you need:
10.

- A Clean and Clear Glass Jar with a Lid
- A Wide-Mouthed Jug
- A Muslin Bag
- A Dark Glass Bottle
- A Funnel
- Herbs
- Oil

To infuse herbal oil the cold way, follow these steps:

1. Place dried herbs in a sterilized jar. For a decent batch, add about 500 g (17.6 oz) of herbs.
2. Pour about 2 cups of olive oil over the herbs.
3. Close the jar, securing tightly, and give it a few good shakes.
4. Place the jar someplace sunny, like a windowsill, and let it sit for two to six weeks. Shake occasionally.

5. Place the muslin bag over the jug, securing it over the rim and tucking the middle of the cloth inside.

6. Pour the oil through the muslin, and bring the edges of the cloth together, trapping the herbs inside. Keep squeezing until all the liquid is strained.

7. With the help of a funnel, pour the strained oil into a dark glass bottle. Use as needed.

*Dosage*: Unless the herbs used come with special precautions or concerns about your unique condition, you should be free to apply or consume the oil as much as you think is necessary.

*Storage*: Store the bottles somewhere dry and dark for up to one year. For best results, make a habit of using the oil within six months, as after that the oil will start losing its medicinal powers.

*Note*: So, keep in mind that most herbs work well dried but a few need to be used fresh. That is one reason you need to know your plant. Some Herbs need to be fresh when the oil is added, because, their oils need to be infused in the carrier oil instead of evaporating. For instance, dried lemon had some value for relieving depression but not much value against Herpes virus unless fresh. Much of its medicinal value is in the plant's oils. If you make the infused oil with fresh herb, it has multiple uses instead of limited uses.

If you are unsure about your herbs or the procedures, you are very welcome to join our private herbal community in Facebook and get advice from other herbalists. You will find the QR code at the end of this book. You scan the QR code with your camera and it takes you to our group. You can also just search "Herbalism For Beginners At Home - Medicinal Herbs and Herbalist Remedies" and request to join our group.

## Essential Oils

In the past, essential oils were where I drew the line. I could whip up creams, tinctures and infusions, but making essential oils was something I always steered away from. That is until I developed the confidence to give it a try! Homemade essential oils are not only cost effective, especially if you have an herb garden, but they can also be very rewarding to make. There is something empowering about being able to say, "Here, try the essential oil I've made."

As challenging as the process may sound, it is actually very simple. If you think about it, essential oils are no more than products distilled from steam. You just simmer the herb, the steam goes through a tube, the tube runs through cold water, condensation occurs, and that's it. Your essential oil is born.

And you don't need tons of fancy ingredients either. You can do it with just a few essentials:

- A Crockpot with a Lid
- Distilled Water
- 3–4 cups of Fresh Herbs
- Small Dark Glass Bottles
- A Turkey Baster
- A Stove

Ready to give it a try? Here are the steps to making your first essential oil:

1. Chop up your preferred herbs, using enough to fill the crockpot about ¾ of the way. Usually, about 3–4 cups of plant material should suffice.
2. Pour enough distilled water into the crockpot to cover the chopped herbs.
3. Place the lid on but put it <u>upside down</u>. This is important, as the lid's concave curves will push the steam back inside. Alternatively, you can use a plate for this purpose.
4. Place the crockpot over high heat and cook until the water becomes very hot. Then turn the heat to low and allow the herbs to simmer for a good three to four hours.
5. Remove from heat and allow to cool completely.
6. Transfer to the fridge and leave it there overnight.

7. The next day, when uncovering the pot, you will notice that a thin, oily film has formed on top of the liquid. That's your essential oil. This layer will be slightly hardened and you need to gather it quickly as it will soon start to melt away, as the pot warms up to room temperature. For extra precision, use a turkey baster for this step. It will be like lifting excess fat from the top of the gravy. Then fill up your sterilized dark glass bottles.

8. If you don't follow these steps correctly, you might notice some water-based liquid at the bottom of the bottle of essential oil. If this bothers you, you can reheat the oil so that the water will become steam and escape from the bottle. If you do that, be super gentle; essential oils lose their potency when heated, so don't overdo it.

Always use fresh herbs for this extraction method, as the dried versions will contain significantly less essential oil. Chopping the plants is also crucial, to increase the surface area from which oils can escape the herbs.

<u>Storage</u>: Secured tightly, the glass bottles should be stored in a dark and cool place. You can generally use them for up to a year, but after the first six months the essential oils will begin to lose their potency.

## Tonic Wines

Tonic wines are the best way to extract the medicinal properties from tonic herbs, and the most effective method for supporting digestion and improving vitality. Angelica, especially Chinese dong quai angelica, is one of the most popular herbal ingredients for making a red or white wine tonic.

The key to making an especially potent tonic wine is to keep oxygen exposure to a minimum. That is why I don't recommend doing this in bottles, jugs, or pots that will be opened and exposed to the atmosphere regularly. Herbs soaked in wine will turn moldy if they are frequently in contact with air. To prevent this from happening, I suggest using a jar with a tap at the base. That way, you have control over the flow of wine without exposing the mixture to the air or upsetting the herbs.

To make a tonic wine, you will need:

- 1 liter (1 quart) of Red or White Wine
- 100 g (3.5 oz) of Dried Tonic Herbs or 25–30 g (1 oz) of Dried Bitter Herbs
- A Clean Jar with a Tap at the Base

**Steps to making a tonic wine:**

1. Place the dried herbs inside a sterilized jar.
2. Pour the wine over the herbs, keeping in mind that the wine should cover the herbs completely.
3. Close the jar tightly and give it a gentle shake.
4. Let the jar sit for two to six weeks so that the herbs can soak and the wine can become more mature.

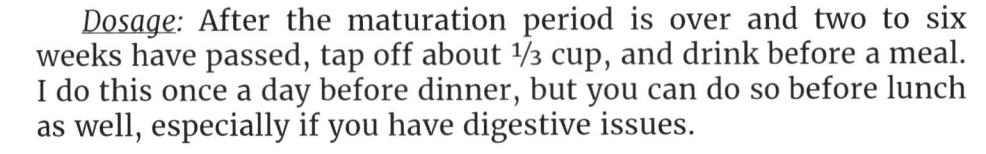

*Dosage:* After the maturation period is over and two to six weeks have passed, tap off about ⅓ cup, and drink before a meal. I do this once a day before dinner, but you can do so before lunch as well, especially if you have digestive issues.

*Storage:* If stored properly, the wine will be safe to consume for at least three months. If the wine takes on a funny flavor and aroma, it may signify that the herbs have become moldy or the wine has oxidized. If that happens, discard the remedy, and steep yourself a new batch.

# Poultices

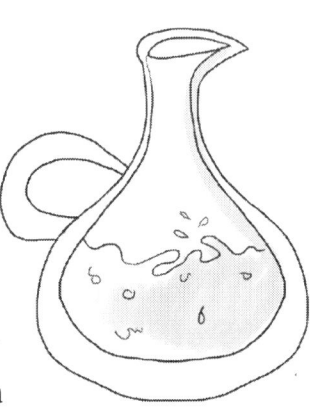

When I'm making poultices, I always feel like a Victorian nurse using my herbalist powers to relieve someone's condition. Once you try your hand at whipping up these soothing mixtures, you will also begin to feel like a herbal healer. As simple as this method is, it can be ten times more effective than other methods we have discussed.

Poultices are a simple mix of fresh, powdered, or dried herbs, simmered and applied to an affected area on the skin. The herbs' active substances will seep through the skin and do their magic to ease nerve or muscle pain and promote healing.

To make your own poultice, you will need:

- A Saucepan
- Some Gauze
- A Little Bit of Water
- A Few Drops of Oil
- A Stove

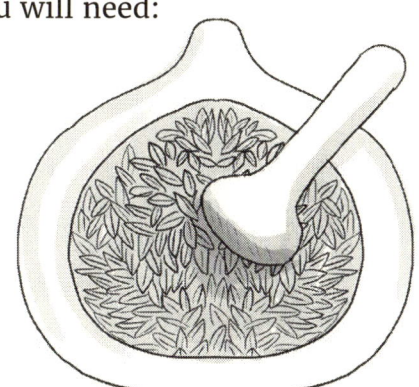

And here is how you can do it:

1. Place your herbs in the saucepan and add a bit of water to the pan. Don't go overboard, but use a sufficient amount. There should be enough water to cover the affected area of your skin.

2. Place saucepan over medium heat and simmer for two to three minutes.

3. Scoop the herbs up with a spoon and carefully squeeze the excess liquid from them. You can do this with a second spoon or by pressing the mixture in your hands.

4. Rub a few drops of oil onto the affected area to prevent the herbs from sticking to the skin.

5. Apply the simmered herbs, while still hot, onto the location, and place the gauze over the top of the herbs, tying it securely to make sure the herbs stay in contact.

6. Leave for two to three hours, or as needed.

*Application:* Every two or three hours, apply a new poultice until the condition's severity subsides.

## Ointments

The thing that makes ointments so effective is that they use fatty ingredients and absolutely no water. These applications can form a protective layer over the skin, which is especially useful when treating inflammation or damaged surfaces. The point is for the ointment to keep moisture at bay, sealing the skin off from water and the environment. This is why ointments are so helpful with treating conditions like diaper rash.

I used to think it was impossible to replace store-bought ointments with homemade herbal remedies, but this recipe for ointment will convince any skeptic otherwise.

Here is what you need:

- A Double Boiler (Or a Saucepan and a Heat-Resistant Bowl)
- Herb-infused Oil of Choice
- Beeswax
- A Wooden Spatula
- Small Dark Glass Jars with Lids

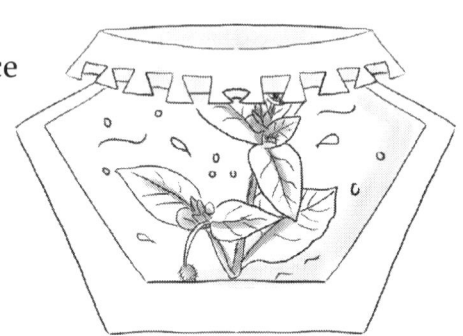

Method of preparation for ointments:

1. Melt wax in double boiler, or in the heat-resistant bowl placed over a saucepan containing warm water.
2. Add oil. Use 1 cup herb-infused oil to 2 tablespoons beeswax.
3. Remove from the heat and stir till cool enough to stay emulsified (combined).
4. Pour into containers and cool completely.

Beeswax can be difficult to clean out of your double boiler and so, to avoid this tiresome problem, I use a small can that I place in a saucepan containing a little warm water. This works in a similar manner to a water bath. The advantage is that, once I have finished working with the beeswax, I leave the remainder in the can to harden. I cover the can and leave it until the next time I wish to make an ointment. This saves contaminating your double boiler with sticky beeswax.

A salve is a thicker version of an ointment. It is made in the same way as described above, but the ratio of beeswax to oil should be 1:2. If you wish, you can use part coconut oil when you make the original herb-infused oil for your ointment or salve. Ointments and salves should stay on top of the skin to protect damaged areas, and the active ingredients should be absorbed into the body for the soothing, pain-relieving properties to have their effect.

*Dosage:* Apply a small amount of the ointment onto the affected area, three times a day. If you are using an ointment to treat diaper rash, apply it with every diaper change.

*Storage:* Store your tightly closed dark glass jars in a cool and dark spot, and use within three months.

## Creams

Unlike ointments that are water-free, creams are mixtures of fat and water. They do not offer a protective layer on the surface but blend with the skin. The medicinal properties provide a cooling or soothing effect. In this way, the skin is allowed to breathe and can heal much more quickly.

I've found that my creams are most beneficial and much gentler when made with a wax and glycerin combination. You could use a traditional glycerite, which is a fluid extract of an herb, made using glycerin as part of the extraction medium. I am sharing my secret recipe with you now.

You will need:

- A Saucepan and Heat-Resistant Glass Bowl, or a Small Double Boiler

- A Wooden Spatula
- A Muslin Bag
- A Jug or Pot
- A Spread Knife
- Small Dark Glass Jars
- Beeswax
- Glycerin and Herbs (or Glycerite of Choice)
- Water

The method:

1. Fill a saucepan half way with water and place over high heat. Bring to a boil.
2. Lower the heat to a simmer and rest a glass bowl over the pan. Or use a double boiler instead.
3. Add about 150 g (5.3 oz) of beeswax to the bowl and stir until melted.
4. Then, stir in the glycerin; about 75 g (2.7 oz), or ½ the amount of wax.
5. Add ⅓ cup of water to the mix.
6. Stir in about 30 g (1.05 oz) of dried herbs and cover the glass bowl.
7. Leave the mixture to heat gently, over the hot water of the saucepan, for three full hours.
8. Secure the muslin bag over a jug or pot and pour the herb mixture through to strain it.
9. Bring the edges of the bag together and squeeze to push the strained liquid into the jug.
10. Stir gently as the mixture cools and the cream sets.
11. Have your sterilized dark glass jars ready and transfer the cream into the jars with the help of a small spread knife.

12. Secure tightly and store in refrigerator until needed.

*Tip:* You can also add extra ingredients to your creams such as powders, tinctures, or essential oils for an added medicinal boost.

*Dosage:* Apply the cream to the affected area up to three times a day.

*Storage:* Unlike ointments, creams deteriorate quickly due to the water content. They should be stored in the fridge. If secured tightly, they should last for a good three months.

## Compresses

After my usual hiking misadventures and clumsiness, I often come home with a swollen ankle or a particularly bruised knee. After returning, I take a relaxing shower, put my leg up, apply a compress onto the affected area, and enjoy a cup of herbal infusion or tea.

A compress is just a cloth that has been soaked in an herbal infusion or decoction, and then applied onto an injury or bruise to promote healing or alleviate pain.

To make a compress, you will need:

- A Clean Bowl
- Clean Soft Cloth or Washcloth
- Infusion, Decoction or Tincture and Water Mix

Method for preparing a compress:

1. Prepare your infusion or decoction, strain well, and let it cool so it is not unbearably hot. For a compress, you will need about 2 cups of infusion or decoction. You can also make this with a tincture. If you are using a tincture, combine 5 tsp of tincture in 2 cups of water.

2. Pour the infusion, decoction or diluted tincture into a clean bowl.

3. Soak the clean cloth completely in the infused liquid, then wring out the excess.

4. Place the soaked cloth onto the affected area. You can even secure it with some safety pins or string.

5. Re-soak as it cools and replace. The warmth will feel good and improve the absorption of the herb(s).

6. Leave for one to two hours.

Instead of applying the compress, you can also use a lotion bath for the same purpose. Instead of placing the cloth over the area after wringing out the excess liquid, just wring out the liquid directly over the affected area. Soak, wring, bathe, repeat. Soon, you will have the desired results.

*Application*: Use as needed.

*Storage:* Store the compress infusions in clean bottles in the fridge for up to 48 hours.

## Powders, Capsules, Pills

Powdered herbs are just that – herbs that have been ground to a powdered consistency. Usually, a mortar and pestle are used for making powders, but anything that can finely grind can be used for this purpose. Although powders can be sprinkled over food as spices, or even taken with water, one of the most convenient ways to consume an herbal supplement is in capsule form, or rolled into pills.

However, not all herbs can be finely powdered at home. Some may require a more forceful approach; for such herbs, I suggest buying the powdered versions. Most herbal suppliers should be well-stocked with powdered herbs. For making capsules, I recommend looking for a very fine grade of powdered herbs. You will also need empty capsules, which are sold in both gelatin and vegetarian form, in most specialist outlets.

To make capsules you will need:

– A Saucer

- Powdered Herbs
- Empty Capsules

And this is how you can make capsules:

1. Pour the powdered herb into a saucer.
2. Holding two empty capsule halves, scoop the powder up by sliding the capsule halves towards each other.
3. Once you have filled the capsule cases, gently slide them together, keeping the powder locked inside.

For a 00-size capsule, you will need about 250 mg of powder. If this is something you decide to do often, you could consider purchasing a small machine that will help you fill many capsules in a short time; also, it packs the powdered herb so tightly that a 00-size capsule holds up to 450 mg.

*Dosage:* Depending on the herb used, take two to three capsules a day.

*Storage:* Place the capsules in dark glass containers and store them in a dark and cool place for up to three or four months.

To make pills you will need:

- A Small Bowl
- Powdered Herbs
- Binding Agent such as Honey or Gum Tragacanth
- Oven

And this is how you can make your own pills:

1. Pour your powdered herbs into the small bowl.
2. Add a teaspoon of honey (or other binding agent) and enough water to make a paste that resembles bread dough.
3. Roll out into the shape of a long, thin rope.
4. Cut the rope into small segments. (You can now roll each segment in a powdered spice of your choice, such as cin-

namon.)

5. Place the pills onto a baking tray and dry them in a cool oven.

*Dosage*: Depending on the herb used, take two to three pills a day.

*Storage*: The pills should be stored in a dry and cool place in a dark glass jar up to four months.

## Steam Inhalations

Steam inhalations are my go-to remedy for the sinus-related troubles caused by seasonal allergies. These inhalations are an effective way to clear congestion, especially when using herbs that have antiseptic medical actions, such as goldenseal, thyme, or myrrh.

To make a steam inhalation, you will need:

- 25–30 g (1 oz) of Preferred Herbs
- 1 Liter of Water (1 Quart)
- A Pot
- A Towel
- A Stove

And the method for creating a steam inhalation is quite simple:

1. Heat the water to a boil before pouring over the herb leaves or flowers.
2. Allow to steep for 15 minutes.
3. If you are using roots or barks, which release their goodies when simmered, you should simmer for 15 minutes, then allow cool for a further 15 minutes.
4. Reheat liquid to simmer (a bit cooler than a boil).

5. Remove the pot from the heat.

6. Place your head over the pot, and cover both your head and the bowl with the towel.

7. Close your eyes, and stay in this position, inhaling steam for approximately ten minutes.

Remember that high heat destroys the value in many herbs; I recommend to never boil herbs, but to just simmer them. I strongly advise you not to rush the process of using a steam inhalation. If you're impatient like me, you can put on some music to help you relax. I also recommend not leaving the room for about 15 minutes, even after the inhalation process is complete. This is so that you can further support the clearing of congestion.

## Mouth Gargles and Washes

Mouthwashes and gargles are usually used to treat infections and inflammation of the mouth and throat. They are most effective with herbs that have astringent compounds, such as myrrh, as they can heal and repair the mucous membrane. To make them more beneficial for the throat, you can also add a small amount of licorice to the mix.

To make a mouthwash or gargle, you will need:

- ⅓ Cup of Infusion
- A Glass

And here is how you do it:

1. Make an infusion with your preferred herbs, but do not strain right away. To increase the astringency, let the herbs sit in the saucepan for about 15 minutes longer.

2. Strain, as you normally would, and pour into a glass, only filling the glass about ⅓ of the way.

3. Gargle or rinse the mouth with small portions of the liquid.

The best thing about these homemade herbal gargles and mouthwashes is that they are made with natural and safe ingredients through infusion or decoction. This means that you don't need to worry about accidentally swallowing the liquid. On the contrary, doing so can further benefit your health.

*Tip: You can also make a mouthwash by mixing 1/3 cup of hot water and 1 tsp (about 5 ml) of your preferred tincture.*

Each of the above preparation methods allows healing substances in the herbs to be extracted differently and also results in different ways of applying the extract. While you can use an infusion for drinking, gargling, or placing onto an affected area as a compress, there is only one way of applying an ointment.

Before using any of these methods to address a health concern, make sure to inform yourself of the possible risks and side effects. While a syrup may present some benefit, that may not be the best application for your mouth sores. Similarly, a tincture of myrrh may not be helpful for your insomnia.

The next chapters will teach you all about pairing particular conditions with the right remedies, thereby removing all the guesswork involved in becoming a master of herbal healing.

# 71 Ailments and Their Herbal Remedies

Herbal remedies can be a safer, more natural, and even a healthier alternative to conventional medication. Their effects depend on the condition's intensity and other factors that are unique to each individual; generally, herbs provide a powerful and efficient healing base. Some ailments may need a chemical approach, of course, but for most health issues, the cure lies in nature. Here are the most common 71 health concerns that can be treated easily with natural, plant-based remedies. For each ailment, I have suggested only a small sample of the many different herbs that can be used for treatment. There are many other remedies out there and each human body reacts best to a certain remedy. You will get to know what works best for your body by experimenting with different herbs, one at a time.

### #1 Anemia
Herb: Nettle
Remedy: Make nettle infusion and drink 3 cups a day.

### #2 Anxiety
Herb: Valerian, Hops
Remedies: Add about 10 drops of valerian tincture into water and drink, a couple of times a day, for two weeks. For excessive anxiety, make a hops tincture and dilute 20 drops of the tincture into a glass of water. Take this mixture up to six times a day.

### #3 Acne
Herbs:

Calendula, Comfrey, Echinacea

Remedies: Calendula and comfrey cream can be applied to the affected area twice a day. In addition, you can consume one echinacea tablet a day for several weeks.

### #4 Allergies
Herbs: Nettle, Elderflower

Remedies: Take 1–2 cups of a nettle infusion each day for three months; or use 1 cup elderflower infusion each day, starting one month before the hay fever season, and continuing for its duration.

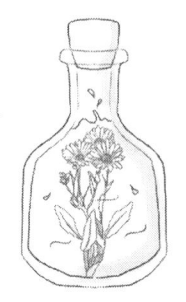

### #5 Asthma
Herb: Echinacea, Nettle, Thyme

Remedies: For shortness of breath, concoct a nettle and thyme infusion, and take about 3 cups a day; for mild bronchial asthma, make echinacea tablets and take one daily.

### #6 Athlete's Foot
Herbs: Turmeric, Calendula

Remedy: Make a calendula ointment and combine 3 tsp of the ointment with ½ tsp of turmeric powder. Rub the affected area daily.

### #7 Backache
Herbs: St. John's Wort, Lavender, Rosemary, Thyme

Remedies: Make 3 cups of a thyme infusion, add to the warm water in a bath, and soak for 20 minutes; combine 20 drops of lavender essential oil, 2 tbsp St. John's Wort infused oil, and 10 drops of rosemary essential oil, and rub into the tense area.

### #8 Bee Sting
Herbs: Lavender, Nettle

Remedy: Rub nettle leaf on the sting area (after removing the stinger) or apply lavender essential oil or tincture, for relief.

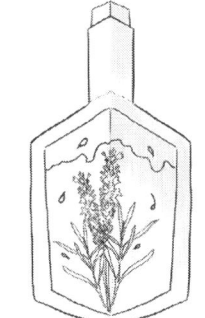

### #9 Bloating
Herbs: Fennel, Peppermint

Remedies: Make a fennel infusion by combining ½ tsp of fennel seeds and ¾ cup of water. Drink this infusion three times a day; or consume 1 cup of a peppermint infusion one to three times a day.

## #10 Bronchitis
Herb: Echinacea
Remedy: Combine ½ tsp of echinacea tincture with some water, and drink two to three times a day. Alternatively, you can take one echinacea tablet daily.

## #11 Bruises
Herbs: Arnica
Remedy: Apply an arnica ointment onto the affected area two to three times a day, but only if the skin is not broken.

## #12 Burns
Herbs: Aloe Vera, Lavender, Calendula
Remedies: Apply aloe vera gel or lavender essential oil onto the affected area after the heat is gone. Repeat as needed. Make a calendula infusion and apply it cold onto the affected area.

## #13 Chapped Lips
Herb: Elderflower
Remedy: Make a cream or ointment from elderflowers and apply the mixture onto chapped lips. It should work well on any chapped surface of your skin.

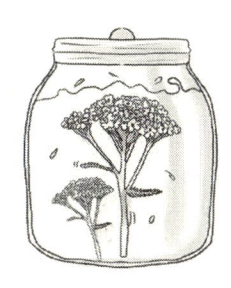

## #14 Canker Sore
Herb: Myrrh
Remedy: Combine ½ tsp of myrrh tincture with 3 tsp of water and gargle for one minute.

## #15 Chickenpox
Herbs: Echinacea, St. John's Wort, Lemon Balm
Remedy: Take about half a teaspoon of echinacea tincture with some water, and drink it a couple of times a day. This will boost the immune system. In addition, take half a teaspoon of lemon balm tincture, or make a salve with lemon balm oil. Lemon balm is particularly successful against the virus that causes chickenpox. Lastly, half a teaspoon of St. John's wort tincture in water, or a cream made with St. John's wort tincture, will help soothe itching and pain.

### #16 Cold
Herb: Ginger
Remedy: Infuse 3 slices of fresh ginger in ¾ cup of water. Drink three times a day.

### #17 Cold Sore
Herb: Lemon Balm
Remedies: Make a lemon balm Infusion and sip throughout the day, consuming no more than 3 cups. You can also infuse 3 tsp of fresh or freshly dried lemon balm in ¾ cup water for ten minutes to use externally. Strain, let cool and then dab onto the affected area three times a day.

### #18 Colic
Herb: Fennel
Remedy: Combine 1 level tsp of fennel seeds and ¾ cups of water. Simmer for ten minutes, strain, allow to cool slightly and offer to your baby. It is healthy to drink up to one cup per day.

### #19 Conjunctivitis
Herb: German Chamomile
Remedy: Infuse two German Chamomile tea bags in two cups of water. Allow to cool, squeeze out the excess tea, and place the teabags over the eyes.

### #20 Constipation
Herbs: Peppermint, Ginger, Dandelion, Licorice
Remedies: Teas and infusions made from any combination of the herbs mentioned above can be powerful for battling constipation. Drink 2–3 cups a day.

### #21 Cough
Herb: Thyme
Remedy: Make a thyme infusion and consume 3 cups a day.

### #22 Dandruff
Herb: Tea Tree
Remedy: Dilute a few drops of tea tree essential oil in your regular shampoo, and wash your hair as usual. Do not apply tea tree oil undiluted directly on the scalp. This usage can cause in-

flammation and rashes.

### #23 Diaper Rash
<u>Herbs</u>: Chickweed, Calendula
<u>Remedies</u>: Make chickweed ointment and apply once or twice a day. Calendula ointment can be applied to dry skin each time you're changing a diaper.

### #24 Diarrhea
<u>Herb</u>: Agrimony
<u>Remedy</u>: Drink about 1 ½ cups of an agrimony infusion each day for three days.

### #25 Digestive Inflammation Including GERD (Gastroesophageal Reflux Disease)
<u>Herb</u>: Licorice
<u>Remedy</u>: Make a licorice tincture and combine ½ tsp of this tincture with ½ cup of water. Drink twice a day.

### #26 Earache
<u>Herb</u>: Lavender, Garlic, Mullein
<u>Remedy</u>: Place a couple of drops of lavender essential oil onto a cotton ball and place it inside the affected ear as a plug. Keep the cotton ball in place for at least 10–15 minutes. Garlic-Mullein ear oil is an even more effective remedy, used in the same way. Do not drop undiluted essential oils directly into the ear canal.

### #27 Eczema
<u>Herb</u>: German Chamomile, Witch Hazel
<u>Remedies</u>: Make about 3 cups of chamomile infusion. Add this infusion to a bath while it is still hot, and soak for 15–25 minutes. You can also allow the infusion to cool and apply it to the itchy area as a compress. You can also use a witch hazel cream, applying it to the affected area up to five times a day.

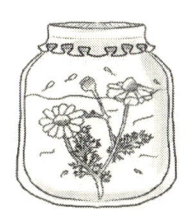

### #28 Fatigue
<u>Herbs</u>: Ginseng, St. John's Wort
<u>Remedies</u>: Make ginseng capsules and take up to 1 g of powder a day. Make a St. John's wort infusion and consume no more than 2⅓ cups a day.

### #29 Fever
Herbs: Yarrow, Elderberry
Remedy: Infuse ½ tsp each of yarrow and elderberry in ⅓ cup of water. Brew for ten minutes and drink five to six times a day. Do not consume more than 2⅓ cups a day.

### #30 Flu
Herbs: Thyme, Elderflower, Lemon Balm
Remedy: Place about 1½–2 tbsp of each herb in 3 cups of water. Brew for ten minutes and drink up. Do not consume more than 3 cups a day.

### #31 Fractures
Herb: Comfrey
Remedies: Make comfrey ointment or cream, and apply these mixtures to the affected area, three to four times a day, as long as the skin is not broken. Alternatively, you can make a comfrey infusion and apply cold compresses to the area.

### #32 Gastritis
Herb: Goldenseal
Remedies: Make goldenseal capsules with goldenseal powder and take one, three times a day. Alternatively, you can drink 2 cups of goldenseal infusion daily. Note that this can be VERY bitter.

### #33 Gingivitis (Gum Inflammation)
Herb: Myrrh
Remedy: Using the same remedy as was used for canker sores, combine ½ tsp of myrrh tincture and 3 tsp of water, and gargle for a minute.

### #34 Hair Loss
Herb: Thyme
Remedy: Make a thyme infusion, allow to cool, and massage the warm mixture into the scalp to reverse hair loss and support hair growth.

### #35 Halitosis (Bad Breath)
Herb: Tea Tree, Sage
Remedy: Dilute one drop of tea tree oil in a couple of vegetable oil drops and add it to a cup of warm water. Rinse your mouth

with some of the solution for 30 seconds and spit out. Do this until you have used the entire cup. Alternatively, make 1 cup of sage Infusion, rinse your mouth with some of the solution for 30 seconds and spit out. Rinse and repeat until the cup is empty.

### #36 Hangover
Herb: Dandelion
Remedy: Make a decoction with 15 g (½ oz) of dandelion root and 3 cups of water. Drink, in small quantities, frequently during the day.

### #37 Headache
Herbs: Rosemary, Lavender
Remedies: Make a rosemary infusion and drink 2 cups a day. As a general headache remedy, you can also rub lavender or rosemary essential oil on the temples for a couple of minutes to relax and calm the pain in your head.

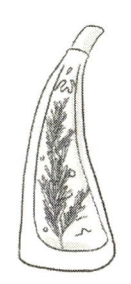

### #38 Hemorrhoids
Herb: Witch Hazel
Remedy: Apply witch hazel ointment after each bowel movement, or once to twice a day.

### #39 High Blood Pressure
Herbs: Garlic, Ginkgo
Remedies: Eat one to two fresh garlic cloves each day, or take one garlic tablet daily. As an alternative, take one ginkgo tablet a day for two to three months

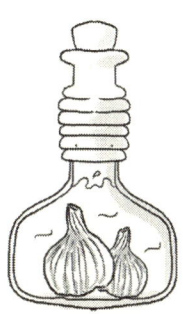

### #40 Hives
Herbs: Chickweed, Nettle
Remedies: Apply chickweed cream to the affected area or make a nettle infusion and drink it regularly throughout the day, consuming no more than 3 cups in total.

### #41 Indigestion
Herb: German Chamomile, Fennel
Remedy: Make a chamomile, or a fennel seed infusion and drink 1 cup after each meal, or as needed.

### #42 Insect Bites
Herbs: Sage, Basil, Thyme
Remedy: Extract the juice from the leaves of one of the herbs above and apply directly onto the bites.

### #43 Insomnia
Herbs: Lavender, Chamomile, Valerian
Remedies: Make a lavender infusion and drink ¾ cup before bedtime. Alternatively, take 1 cup of chamomile infusion before going to bed. For a more intense state of insomnia, make valerian tablets, and take one before going to bed.

### #44 Liver Infections
Herb: Milk Thistle
Remedy: Make a milk thistle decoction and drink about ⅓ cup a day.

### #45 Menopause
Herbs: Sage, Black Cohosh
Remedies: Make a sage infusion and drink one cup at night to reduce night sweats and hot flashes. In addition, you can also take one black cohosh tablet to tackle fluctuating estrogen and progesterone levels.

### #46 Mental Focus
Herb: Ginkgo
Remedy: Make ginkgo tablets and take one daily.

### #47 Muscle Cramps
Herb: Arnica
Remedy: Make an arnica cream or ointment, and apply it to the affected area, massaging for a minute or two.

### #48 Nausea
Herb: Lemon Balm
Remedy: Make a lemon balm infusion using dried herbs and drink 2–3 cups a day.

### #49 Period Pain
Herb: Black Cohosh
Remedy: Make a black cohosh tincture and combine 40 drops of this mixture with ½ cup of water. Drink three times a day.

## #50 Premenstrual Syndrome (PMS)
Herbs: Vervain, Rosemary
Remedies: Make vervain tablets and take one daily. Add 5–10 drops of rosemary essential oil to a bath and soak for twenty minutes.

## #51 Psoriasis
Herb: Turmeric
Remedy: Make a poultice with 1 tsp of turmeric powder and a just enough water to form a paste. Apply directly to the affected area, three times a day. Be careful as turmeric stains, especially clothes.

## #52 Rheumatoid Arthritis
Herb: Black Cohosh
Remedy: Make a black cohosh decoction, and sip throughout the day, consuming up to 3 cups each day.

## #53 Shingles
Herbs: Garlic, Ginger, Lemon Balm
Remedies: Apply fresh ginger or garlic slices onto unopened shingles up to six times a day. Make a lemon balm infusion and drink 2–3 cups daily. Alternatively, a salve made with lemon balm can be applied to the shingles and this will help fight the virus that causes the condition.

## #54 Sinus Infection
Herb: German Chamomile, Thyme
Remedy: Make a steam inhalation with 15 g (½ ounce) of chamomile or thyme in 3 cups of water. Place your head over the pot with the infusion, throw a towel over both your head and the pot, and inhale for ten minutes.

## #55 Skin Tags
Herb: Tea Tree
Remedy: Add a few drops of tea tree essential oil to a cotton ball and apply it onto the skin tag, letting it rest there for about ten minutes. A piece of sticking plaster will help to keep it in place. Do this three times a day for as long as it takes for the tag to fall off.

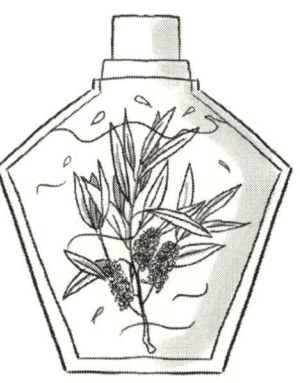

### #56 Sore Muscles
<u>Herbs</u>: Thyme, Rosemary
<u>Remedy</u>: Make 3 cups of infusion with one (or both) of the herbs and add the hot water to a bath. Soak for about 20 minutes.

### #57 Sore Throat
<u>Herbs</u>: Rosemary, Myrrh, Echinacea
<u>Remedy</u>: Add ⅓ tsp of each herb to 5 tsp of warm water, mix to combine, and gargle for a minute. Do not swallow if pregnant.

### #58 Sprains
<u>Herb</u>: Arnica, Comfrey
<u>Remedy</u>: Make arnica cream or ointment, apply to the affected area, and massage in for a few minutes. Do this three times a day. Make a comfrey poultice and apply to the sprain.

### #59 Stiff Joints
<u>Herbs</u>: St. John's Wort, Lavender
<u>Remedy</u>: Combine about 2 ½ tbsp of St. John's wort-infused oil with 20–30 drops of lavender essential oil and massage the mixture into the stiff area.

### #60 Stomach Spasms
<u>Herbs</u>: German Chamomile, Angelica
<u>Remedy</u>: Make an infusion with three parts of chamomile and one part of angelica root. Sip throughout the day, consuming up to 3 cups.

### #61 Stress
<u>Herb</u>: Ginseng
<u>Remedy</u>: Take one to two ginseng capsules a day.

### #62 Sunburn
<u>Herb</u>: Aloe Vera
<u>Remedy</u>: Apply aloe vera gel to the sunburned area as often as necessary.

### #63 Swelling and Fluid Retention
<u>Herb</u>: Dandelion
<u>Remedies</u>: Make dandelion leaf infusion and drink 2 cups a day. You can also make dandelion juice from the

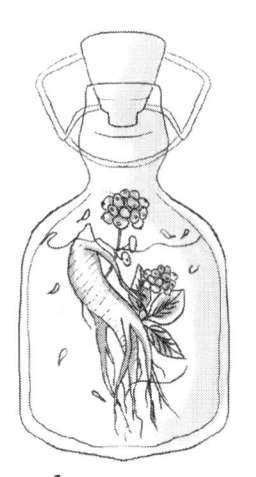

leaves of the plant, and consume 1 tbsp of the juice three times a day.

### #64 Tongue Ulcers
Herbs: Myrrh, Licorice, Echinacea
Remedies: Combine equal parts of the tinctures of the herbs and apply neatly onto the area of the mouth. Alternatively, dilute one part of the tincture mixture in five parts water and gargle.

### #65 Tonsillitis
Herb: Echinacea
Remedy: Make echinacea tablets and take one to two each day. Take no more than 1 g of powder a day.

### #66 Travel Sickness
Herbs: Ginger, Turmeric
Remedy: Make an infusion with 2 slices of ginger and ½ tsp of turmeric powder in ¾ cup of water. Drink no more than 3 cups a day. Alternatively, eat candied ginger, or the powdered ginger spice in your kitchen!

### #67 Urinary Tract Infection (UTI)
Herbs: Garlic, Echinacea
Remedy: Make tablets or capsules of either or both herbs and take one each day.

### #68 Varicose Veins
Herbs: Calendula, Witch Hazel
Remedy: Combine equal parts of calendula and witch hazel cream and apply to the affected area.

### #69 Warts
Herb: Aloe Vera, Tea Tree
Remedy: Apply aloe vera gel onto the wart a couple of times a day for up to three months. You can also dilute 1–2 drops of tea tree essential oil in 12 drops of almond oil, and apply 3–4 drops of the mixture to a cotton ball that you place on the wart. Repeat two or three times a day.

### #70 Wounds
Herbs: Comfrey, Aloe Vera
Remedy: Make comfrey ointment and apply around the edges

of the wounded area. Once you see that a scab has formed, cleanse with aloe vera gel.

### #71 Yeast Infection

<u>Herb</u>: Calendula

<u>Remedy</u>: Make 3 cups of calendula infusion and add, while still warm, to a bath. Soak for 15–25 minutes.

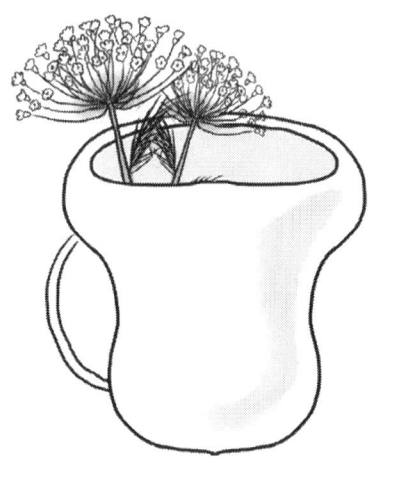

# Handy Herbal Recipes and Mixtures

Although we have already covered 15 extraction methods that can be used to prepare all types of herbal cures, and been through a whopping 71 remedies that will help with the process of healing, it would be remiss not to treat you to some herbal recipes. Think of this chapter as your final lesson in becoming a master herbal healer, in which you finish off your training and invoke your strengths. This final chapter should inspire you to be bold and make your own colorful herbal creations.

## Rosemary and Ginger Tea With Lemon to Strengthen Your Immune System

Ingredients:
1 Slice of Lemon
1 tbsp Sliced Fresh Ginger
1 tsp Chopped Rosemary
1 cup Water

Method:
1. Combine the ginger and water in a small pot, and place over medium heat.

2. Simmer for about five minutes to decoct, then turn off the heat.

3. Add the rosemary and cover the pot. Allow to infuse for ten minutes.

4. Strain the mixture and squeeze the lemon juice into the pot just before serving. Enjoy!

## Tea for Reduced Heart Rate and Lower Blood Pressure

Ingredients:
1 ⅓ tbsp Dried Nettle Leaves
1 ⅓ tbsp Dried Elderberry
1 ⅓ tbsp Dried Lemon Balm
1 ⅓ tbsp Dried Hawthorne Berries
1 liter (1 quart) of Water

Method:
1. Bring the water to a boil and remove the pot from heat.
2. Add the herbs to the pot, and cover.
3. Let sit for five minutes, then strain into a clean bottle.
4. Drink about 3 tbsp of the tea approximately every hour or so for 12 days straight.

## Weight-Loss Tea

Ingredients:
1 tbsp Dried Nettle Leaves
½ tbsp Dried Orange Peel
½ tbsp Sliced Ginger
½ tbsp Dried Dandelion Leaves
¼ tbsp Fennel Seeds
2 ½ cups Water

Method:
1. Bring 2 ½ cups of water to a boil, then remove from heat.
2. Add the herbs, cover the pot, and let sit for three to five minutes.
3. Strain into a bottle and consume during the day.

## Mental Relief Tincture

Ingredients:
1 liter (1 quart) Vodka
5 tbsp Dried Valerian Root
2 tbsp Chopped Rosemary
1 tbsp Chopped Peppermint

Method:
1. Place all the ingredients in a sterilized jar.
2. Seal the jar well and shake to combine.
3. Place in a dark and cool spot and allow to sit for three weeks. Make sure to shake the jar well once a day.
4. Start with ¼ of a tablespoon mixed with some water, and then take additional doses after 30 minutes if needed.

## Ginger and Elderberry Tonic for Winter Vitality

Ingredients:
2 cups Water
1 cup Dried Elderberries
1 tbsp Grated Fresh Ginger
½ cup Raw Honey
1 tsp of Your Favorite Spice (Cinnamon works well for me)

Method:
1. Place the ginger, elderberries, and water in a pot.
2. Place over medium heat and bring just barely to a boil.
3. Reduce the heat to low, then allow the mixture to simmer for 20 minutes or so.
4. Allow to cool until safe to handle and strain the liquid through a sieve.
5. Stir in the honey and spice and pour into a clean glass jar or bottle.
6. Store in the fridge and enjoy 1 tablespoon a day.

## Mouth Wash Mixture (Perfect for Inflammation)

Ingredients:
1 tbsp Dried St. John's Wort
1 tbsp Dried Nettle
1 tbsp Dried Chamomile
¾ liter (¾ quart) Boiling Water

Method:

1. Place the herbs in a small pot and pour the boiling water over them.
2. Cover and let sit for five minutes.
3. Strain the mixture into a clean glass jar or bottle with a lid.
4. Gargle before and after each meal.

**Herb-Infused Massage Oil**

Ingredients:
⅓ cup Fresh Calendula
⅓ cup Fresh St. John's Wort
⅓ cup Fresh Lavender
300 ml (about 10–11 oz) of a Carrier Oil such as Almond, Sesame or Coconut Oil.

Method:
1. Place the plant material inside a previously sterilized glass jar.
2. Pour the carrier oil over the herbs, making sure to leave about two fingers of space for the fresh herbs to expand. The herbs should be totally submerged; otherwise, mold may form.
3. Seal the jar and let it sit in a warm space (near a window is perfect) for 30–40 days.
4. Strain the oil through a cheesecloth and into a clean bottle.
5. Store the massage oil in a dark and cool place, and use it as needed.

**Calendula and Lavender Hand Salve**

Ingredients:
1 tbsp Dried Calendula
1 tbsp Dried Lavender
50–60 ml (2 oz) Coconut Oil
80–90 ml (3 oz) Olive Oil
50–60 g (2 oz) Shea Butter
50–60 g (2 oz) Beeswax Pellets

Method:
1. Place the coconut oil and olive oil in a small pot over medium heat and heat until completely melted. Remove from the heat.

2. Add the calendula and lavender, give the mixture a gentle stir, and let the herbs sit for half an hour to infuse.

3. Strain the oil through cheesecloth or a fine-mesh sieve, into a glass jar.

4. Place the shea butter and beeswax in the pot you used earlier and melt the mixture over medium heat.

5. Add the mixture to the infused oil and stir gently to combine.

6. Seal the jar and let the salve solidify completely before using.

# Stay Safe

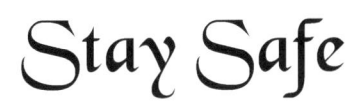

Herbal medicine is indeed safe and natural, but that doesn't mean that it should be approached with no precautions. Not all herbs are harmless, and not all of us have the same health and nutritional requirements. The herbal remedy's effect depends on the active constituents in the herbs and how they interact with your metabolism and your unique medical condition.

Obviously, we cannot possibly cover every minor health issue and discuss every single chemical found in herbs. However, there are general guidelines that each aspiring herbalist must know to ensure safe and effective treatments.

**Stick to What You Know.** Experimenting with herbs you haven't used before is not only unwise, but it can also have a catastrophic effect. Even if you are not allergic to the plant or the herb is generally safe to consume, there may still be severe side effects. Herbs interact with each other and with commercial medications, and can worsen certain conditions. Research the herb well, and make sure that your physical and emotional state can benefit from its use. Also, when trying new treatments, try one herb at a time in case you react to it. If you use a combination, you won't be able to identify which herb disagrees with you.

**Consume Only Appropriate Doses.** Even the safest herbs that you have been consuming as tea, your whole life, can prove to have a negative effect if taken in large quantities. The remedies and preparations in this book suggest medicinal doses that shouldn't be exceeded. Before making your own recipe or self-prescribing a remedy, do some research to pinpoint the exact dosages that are appropriate.

**When in Doubt, Avoid.** The toxicity of certain herbs is not to be toyed with. If you are not sure whether you are overusing a concocted potion, or you have any uncertainties regarding the remedy, do not use it.

**Avoid Long-Term Commitments.** There are hundreds of herbs that are extremely safe to use, but only in the short term. Do some research and see just how long you can safely use a certain herb internally and externally. The safest herbs can be used until the symptoms go away, but if there are no improvements after two or three weeks, consult with a professional practitioner.

*Important: Do not determine the dose yourself, and always follow professional advice.*

**Special Precautions for Children.** Although many herbs can be safely offered to children, I strongly suggest not giving herbal remedies to babies under six months, unless your doctor advises otherwise. Be extremely cautious when giving remedies to children, and keep in mind that the dose must be adjusted, as well. See below:

6–12 months: one-tenth adult dose
1–6 years: one-third adult dose
7–12 years: half adult dose

*The perfect ratio for the adult dose is explained in the extraction methods under "Harnessing the Essence of Herbs."*

**Special Precautions for Pregnancy.** During the first trimester, avoid all herbal medicine unless your OB/GYN advises otherwise. Avoid alcohol-based tinctures when pregnant and use only herbs that are absolutely safe while in this condition.

**Special Precautions for Older People.** Older people, especially those over 70 years, have a much slower metabolism. For that reason, it is recommended that they take ¾ of the recommended adult doses.

**Be Careful with Essential Oils.** Never take essential oils internally unless your doctor gives you the green light. When applying topically, it is always best to dilute the oils with a carrier oil (vegetable or almond oil work well) before applying to the affected area.

**Consider Your Condition.** When searching for a remedy that will work for you, you need to take into consideration how you are feeling, how much you weigh, what you are allergic to, and what conditions you wish to treat. Also, keep in mind that herbal remedies are usually NOT a quick fix. Most treat the cause, not the symptoms. And then one must remember that herbs should not be used for more than three months without a break and a re-evaluation. If they're not doing the job, there may be an underlying reason. Consult with a professional to find out what changes should be made.

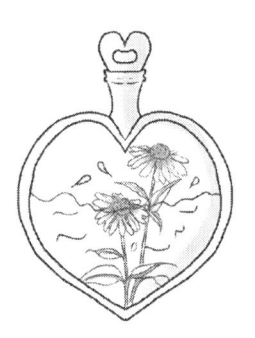

# Conclusion

Congratulations! With the knowledge you've gathered under your belt, you are now officially eligible for trying your hand at some herbal healing.

After learning the basis of herbalism, getting acquainted with 40 of the essential herbs, discovering 15 different extraction methods, and becoming richer with the knowledge of many useful remedies and herbal recipes, it is safe to say that you now have what it takes to become an herbalist. So, feel free to go on a shopping spree for herbalism equipment, plant your herbal garden, and finally whip up plant-based medications for natural healing.

Now the time has come to reach for your mortar and pestle and grab some of your windowsill herbs! Find a simple remedy from this book and see how easy it is when you know what you are doing. From one herbalist to another, I salute your commitment and wish you a well-stocked home apothecary.

Just remember, you do not need much to embark on this journey into therapeutic healing, but you definitely need to travel safely if you want this healing journey to continue.

I'd love to hear all about your herbal adventures! Let's keep in touch! You will find your way to our herbal group below.

# A Small Favor To Ask

## My last request...

Being a smaller author, reviews help me tremendously! **It would mean the world to me** if you could leave a review!

If you liked reading this book and learned a thing or two, please scan the QR with your camera to leave a review!

**Scan with your camera to leave a review!**

Or email "greenhopexllc@gmail.com"
with subject "Thank You Link"
and I will send you the review link and our FB group link!

# Have questions or need advice?
# JOIN our Herbal FAM JAM!

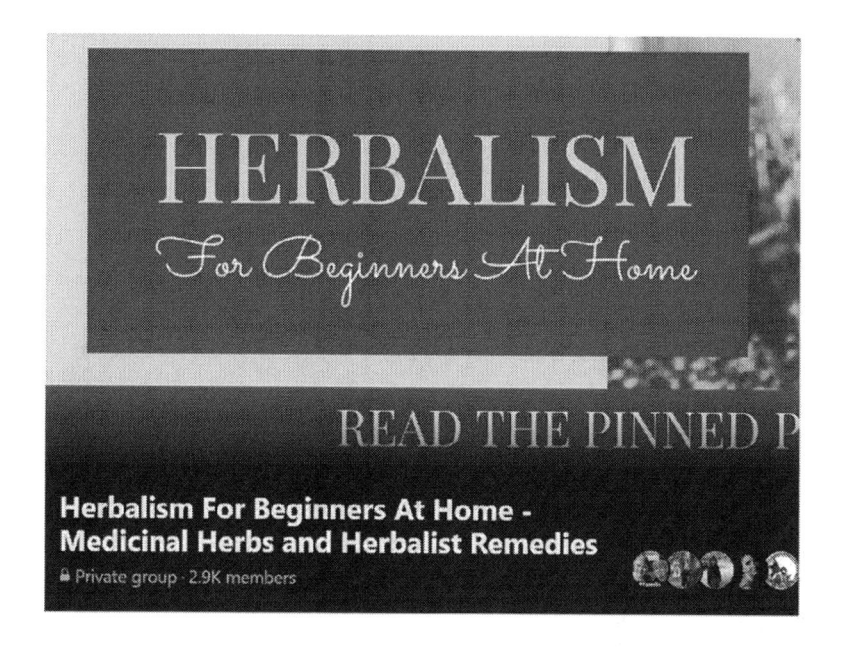

**HERBALISM**
*For Beginners At Home*

READ THE PINNED P

Herbalism For Beginners At Home -
Medicinal Herbs and Herbalist Remedies
Private group · 2.9K members

Connect with like-minded people in our private herbal community on Facebook.

**Scan with your camera to join!**

**Or email "greenhopexllc@gmail.com" with subject "Thank You Link" and I will send you the review link and our FB group link!**

# References and Further Reading

Agrawal, M., Nandini, D., Sharma, V., & Chauhan, N. S. (2010). Herbal remedies for treatment of hypertension. *International Journal of Pharmaceutical Sciences and Research 1* (5), pp. 1–21. http://dx.doi.org/10.13040/IJPSR.0975-8232.1(5).1-21

Alharbi, N. S., Alenizi, A. S., Al-Olayan, A. M., Alobaidi, N. A., Algrainy, A. M., Bahadhailah, A. O., Alhunayni, A. A., Alqurashi, H. D., & Alrohaimi, Y. A. (2018). Herbs use in Saudi children with acute respiratory illnesses. *Sudanese Journal of Paediatrics*, 18(2), 20–24. https://doi.org/10.24911/SJP.106-1538457624

Boadu, A., & Asase, A. (2017). Documentation of herbal medicines used for the treatment and management of human diseases by some communities in southern Ghana. *Evidence-Based Complementary and Alternative Medicine*, Article ID 3043061. https://doi.org/10.1155/2017/3043061

Bodagh, M. N., Maleki, I., & Hekmatdoost, A. (2019). Ginger in gastrointestinal disorders: A systematic review of clinical trials. *Food Science and Nutrition*, 7(5), 96–108. https://doi.org/10.1002/fsn3.807

Chevallier, A. (2016). *Encyclopedia of herbal medicine: 550 Herbs and remedies for common ailments.* Penguin.

Chumpitazi, B. P., Kearns, G. L., & Shulman, R. J. (2018). Review article: the physiological effects and safety of peppermint oil and its efficacy in irritable bowel syndrome and other functional disorders. *Alimentary Pharmacology & Therapeutics*, 47(6), 738–752. https://doi.org/10.1111/apt.14519

CMA. (2012). *A–Z Glossary of terms used in herbal medicine.* The Complementary Medical Association. https://www.the-cma.org.uk/Articles/AZ-Glossary-of-Terms-Used-in-Herbal-Medicine-A-3325/

Daniels, E. (2018). *16 Medicinal plants to keep in your home. ProFlowers.* https://www.proflowers.com/blog/medicinal-plants

Davis, J. (2019). *Harvesting and preserving herbs for the home gardener.* NC State Extension Publication. https://content.ces.ncsu.edu/harvesting-and-preserving-herbs-for-the-home-gardener

Deering, S. (2019). *Nature's 9 most powerful medicinal plants and the science behind them.* Healthline. https://www.healthline.com/health/most-powerful-medicinal-plants

Easley, T., & Horne, S. (2016). *The modern herbal dispensatory: A medicine-making guide.* North Atlantic Books. ISBN:9781623170806.

Ekor, M. (2014). The growing use of herbal medicines: issues relating to adverse reactions and challenges in monitoring safety. *Frontiers in Pharmacology, 4,* p. 177. https://doi.org/10.3389/fphar.2013.00177

Ellis, M. E. (2020). *Turmeric and other anti-inflammatory spices.* Healthline. https://www.healthline.com/health/osteoarthritis/turmeric-and-anti-inflammatory-herbs#garlic

Fisher, M. Z. (2020). *Steam inhalation: How to use fresh herbs to make your own home remedy for congestion relief.* BusinessInsider. https://www.businessinsider.in/science/health/news/steam-inhalation-how-to-use-fresh-herbs-to-make-your-own-home-remedy-for-congestion-relief/articleshow/78838474.cms

Francis, M. (Undated) Healing herbs: Learn to make infused oils and balms. *HGTV Blogsite.* https://www.hgtv.com/design/make-and-celebrate/handmade/diy-herbal-infused-oils

Frost, R., MacPherson, H., & O'Meara, S. (2013). A critical scoping review of external uses of comfrey (*Symphytum* spp.). *Complementary therapies in medicine, 21*(6), 724–745. https://doi.org/10.1016/j.ctim.2013.09.009

Galan, N. (2019). *8 Herbs and supplements for depression.* Medical News Today. https://www.medicalnewstoday.com/articles/314421

Gardner, D. (2002). Evidence-based decisions about herbal products for treating mental disorders. *Journal of Psychiatry and Neuroscience 27*(5): 324–333. https://www.ncbi.nlm.nih.gov/pmc/articles/PMC161674/

Gartrell, E. (2000). More about the Pond's Collection. Rare Book, Manuscript and Special Collections Library, Duke University. https://library.duke.edu/rubenstein/scriptorium/eaa/ponds.html#note

Ghorbanibirgani, A., Khalili, A., & Zamani, L. (2013). The efficacy of stinging nettle (*Urtica dioica*) in patients with benign prostatic hyperplasia: a randomized double-blind study in 100 patients. *Iranian Red Crescent medical journal, 15*(1), 9–10. https://doi.org/10.5812/ircmj.2386

Gladstar, R. (2014). *Herbs for common ailments – how to make and use herbal remedies for home health care.* Storey Publishing. ISBN: 1612124321, 9781612124322.

GI Society. (2008). Time-tested natural remedies for digestive disorders. Canadian Society of Intestinal Research. First published in the *Inside Tract newsletter 165.* https://badgut.org/information-centre/a-z-digestive-topics/time-tested-natural-remedies-for-digestive-disorders/

Hewlings, S. J., & Kalman, D. S. (2017). Curcumin: A review of its effects on human health. *Foods (Basel, Switzerland)*, 6(10), 92. https://doi.org/10.3390/foods6100092

Huizen, J. (2020). *Home and natural remedies for upset stomach.* Medical News Today. https://www.medicalnewstoday.com/articles/322047

Iwanaga, M., Iwanaga, H., Kawakami, N., & World Mental Health Japan Survey Group (2017). Twelve-month use of herbal medicines as a remedy for mental health problems in Japan: A cross-national analysis of World Mental Health Survey data. *Asia-Pacific Psychiatry* 9(3), https://doi.org/10.1111/appy.12285

Jeanroy, E. (2019). How to make herbal infusions. *The Spruce Eats Blogsite.* https://www.thespruceeats.com/how-to-make-an-herbal-infusion-1762142

Johns Cupp, M. (1999). Herbal remedies: Adverse effects and drug interactions. *American Family Physician* 59(5), 1239-1244. https://www.aafp.org/afp/1999/0301/p1239.html

Johnson, T. (2020). *11 Supplements for Menopause.* WebMD. https://www.webmd.com/menopause/ss/slideshow-menopause

Kaur, J., Kaur, S., & Mahajan, A. (2013). Herbal medicine: Possible risks and benefits. *American Journal of Phytomedicine and Clinical Therapeutics* 1(2), 226–239. https://www.imedpub.com/articles/herbal-medicines-possible-risks-andbenefits.pdf

Keiley, L. (2006). *6 Natural Allergy Remedies.* Mother Earth News. https://www.motherearthnews.com/natural-health/natural-allergy-remedies-zmaz06aszraw

Kyrou, I., Christou, A., Panagiotakos, D., Stefanaki, C., Skenderi, K., Katsana, K., & Tsigos, C. (2017). Effects of a hops (*Humulus lupulus* L.) dry extract supplement on self-reported depression, anxiety and stress levels in apparently healthy young adults: A randomized, placebo-controlled, double-blind, crossover pilot study. *Hormones (Athens, Greece)*, 16(2), 171–180. https://doi.org/10.14310/horm.2002.1738

Liang, W., Xu, W., Zhu, J., Zhu, Y., Gu, Q., Li, Y., Guo, C., Huang, Y., Yu, J., Wang, W., Hu, Y., Zhao, Y., Han, B., Bei, W., & Guo, J. (2020). *Ginkgo biloba* extract improves brain uptake of ginsenosides by increasing blood-brain barrier permeability via activating A1 adenosine receptor signaling pathway. *Journal of Ethnopharmacology*, 246, 112243. https://doi.org/10.1016/j.jep.2019.112243

Lu, X., Samuelson, D. R., Rasco, B. A., & Konkel, M. E. (2012). Antimicrobial effect of diallyl sulphide on *Campylobacter jejuni* biofilms. *Journal of Antimicrobial Chemotherapy*, 67(8), 1915–

1926. https://doi.org/10.1093/jac/dks138

Massoud, A., El Sisi, S., Salama, O., & Massoud, A. (2001). Preliminary study of therapeutic efficacy of a new fasciolicidal drug derived from *Commiphora molmol* (myrrh). *The American Journal of Tropical Medicine and Hygiene*, 65(2), 96–99. https://doi.org/10.4269/ajtmh.2001.65.96

Motaleb, M. A., Hossain, M. K., Sobhan, I., Alam, M. K., Khan, N. A., & Firoz, R. (2011) *Selected medicinal plants of Chittagong Hill tracts*. IUCN, Dhaka, Bangladesh. https://www.iucn.org/downloads/medicinal_plant_11_book.pdf

Mulrow, C., Lawrence, V., Jacobs, B., Dennehy, C., Sapp, J., Ramirez, G., Aguilar, C., Montgomery, K., Morbidoni, L., Arterburn, J. M., Chiquette, E., Harris, M., Mullins, D., Vickers, A., & Flora, K. (2000). Milk thistle: Effects on liver disease and cirrhosis and clinical adverse effects; Summary. *AHRQ Evidence Report Summaries*, 21. Rockville (MD): Agency for Healthcare Research and Quality (US); 1998-2005. https://www.ncbi.nlm.nih.gov/books/NBK11896/

Petrovska, B. (2012). Historical review of medicinal plants' usage. *Pharmacognosy Reviews*, 6(11), 1–5. https://doi.org/10.4103/0973-7847.95849

Pittler, M. H., & Ernst, E. (2004). Feverfew for preventing migraine. *The Cochrane Database of Systematic Reviews*, (1), CD002286. https://doi.org/10.1002/14651858.CD002286.pub2

Ratini, M. (2019). *Natural cold and flu remedies*. WebMD. https://www.webmd.com/cold-and-flu/ss/slideshow-natural-cold-and-flu-remedies

Salleh, A. (2014). *Plant chemicals could help Alzheimer's*. ABC Science. URL: https://www.abc.net.au/science/articles/2014/10/15/4098476.htm

Setright, R. (2017). Prevention of symptoms of gastric irritation (GERD) using two herbal formulas: An observational study. *Journal of the Australian Traditional-Medicine Society*, 23(2), 68–71. https://search.informit.org/doi/10.3316/informit.950298610899394 (Original work published June 2017)

Shah, S. A., Sander, S., White, C. M., Rinaldi, M., & Coleman, C. I. (2007). Evaluation of echinacea for the prevention and treatment of the common cold: a meta-analysis. *The Lancet Review*, 7(7), 473-480. https://doi.org/10.1016/S1473-3099(07)70160-3

Shiel, W. Jr. (Undated). *Herbs: Toxicities and drug interactions*. MedicineNet. https://www.medicinenet.com/herbs___toxicities_and_drug_interactions/views.htm

Schrum, C. (2018). *13 Natural remedies for common ailments*. ExperienceLife. https://experiencelife.com/article/13-natural-remedies-for-common-ailments/

Tabassum, N. & Ahmad, F. (2011) Role of natural herbs in the treatment of hypertension. *Pharmacognosy Review* 5(9), pp. 30–40. https://doi.org/10.4103/0973-7847.79097 https://www.ncbi.nlm.nih.gov/pmc/articles/PMC3210006/

Vickers, A., Zollman, C., & Lee, R. (2001). Herbal medicine. *The Western Journal of Medicine*, 175(2), 125–128. https://doi.org/10.1136/ewjm.175.2.125

Widrig, R., Suter, A., Saller, R., & Melzer, J. (2007). Choosing between NSAID and arnica for topical treatment of hand osteoarthritis in a randomised, double-blind study. *Rheumatology International*, 27, 585–591. https://doi.org/10.1007/s00296-007-0304-y

Wikipedia. (2020). *History of herbalism*. Wikipedia. https://en.wikipedia.org/wiki/History_of_herbalism

Wikipedia. (2021). *Medicinal plants*. Wikipedia. https://en.wikipedia.org/wiki/Medicinal_plants

Wolff, H. H., & Kieser, M. (2007). Hamamelis in children with skin disorders and skin injuries: Results of an observational study. *European Journal of Pediatrics*, 166(9), 943–948. https://doi.org/10.1007/s00431-006-0363-1

Wills, R. B. H., Bone, K. & Morgan, M. (2000). Herbal products: Active constituents, modes of action, and quality control. *Nutrition Research Reviews* 13, pp. 47–77. https://www.cambridge.org/core/services/aop-cambridge-core/content/view/8E5D4F8734D795BB107F89E6E5CB8587/S0954422400000044a.pdf/div-class-title-herbal-products-active-constituents-modes-of-action-and-quality-control-div.pdf

Wu, M., Liu, L., Xing, Y., Yang, S., Li, H., & Cao, Y. (2020). Roles and mechanisms of hawthorn and its extracts on atherosclerosis: A review. *Frontiers in Pharmacology*, 11, 118. https://doi.org/10.3389/fphar.2020.00118

Zhang, J., Onakpoya, I. J., Posadzki, P., & Eddouks, M. (2015). The safety of herbal medicine: From prejudice to evidence. *Evidence-Based Complementary and Alternative Medicine*, Article ID 316706. https://doi.org/10.1155/2015/316706

Zick, S. M., Schwabl, H., Flower, A., Chakraborty, B., & Hirschkorn, K. (2009). Unique aspects of herbal whole system research. *Explore (New York)*, 5(2), 97–103. https://doi.org/10.1016/j.explore.2008.12.001

Made in United States
Orlando, FL
27 December 2021